Arthritis

Improve your health,
ease pain, and live
life to the full

Howard Bird, Caroline Green, Andrew Hamer,
Alison Hammond, Janet Harkess, Mike Hurley,
Paula Jeffreson, Dorothy Pattison, David L Scott

London, New York, Munich, Melbourne, Delhi

Senior Editor Janet Mohun
Editor Pip Morgan
Designer Phil Gamble
Senior Art Editor Helen Spencer
Executive Managing Editor Adèle Hayward
Managing Art Editor Karla Jennings
DTP Designer Traci Salter
Picture Researcher Andrea Sadler
Medical Illustrator Philip Wilson
Production Controller Luca Frassinetti

First published in the United Kingdom in 2006 by
Dorling Kindersley Limited, 80 Strand, London WC2R 0RL
A Penguin Company
This paperback edition published in 2009

2 4 6 8 10 9 7 5 3 1

A CIP catalogue record for this book is available from the British Library.
ISBN 978-1-40534-418-0
Reproduced by Colourscan, Singapore
Printed and bound in Singapore by Star Standard

See our complete catalogue at
www.dk.com

Foreword

So many people in the UK have arthritis that you would expect it to be a widely understood condition. After all, it affects about 1 in 5 of us and very few households escape its impact.

Yet myths continue to surround the various forms of the condition: that it affects only older people – the vast majority of those being women – and, most harmfully of all, that there is nothing much you can do about arthritis. As someone who developed arthritis as a boy aged three, and who has worked in this area for decades, I can assure you there is always something you can do about arthritis.

Working out what's going to help you can be the tricky part, though. We are all different and there is no magic formula. What this book allows you to do is to understand arthritis and explore options which might help you or someone else to manage the condition more effectively. The book sets out in simple, plain language what is involved with the various treatments that are available – from the latest therapies to do-it-yourself options like exercise and diet.

There are risks and benefits attached to any response to arthritis and the experts who have contributed to this book describe what these are. Whilst there may be no cure for arthritis, don't let anyone tell you that there is nothing you can do to combat it: quite the opposite is true.

N. J. Betteridge

NEIL BETTERIDGE
CHIEF EXECUTIVE OF ARTHRITIS CARE

Contents

What is arthritis?

In the last 50 years our understanding of arthritis has improved enormously. Where once it was seen as one condition, it is now known to be a group of almost 200. This knowledge has helped doctors to be more specific about diagnosing the type of arthritis and to be able to devise treatments for individual people.

We still don't know what causes arthritis, although we have a much better idea of the risk factors involved – from inheritance and gender to obesity and infections. As a result, we are better placed to know who is likely to develop one or other of the arthritic conditions.

Improvements in diagnosis have gone hand in hand with innovations in scanning techniques, and so arthritis can now be detected earlier and with more precision. Specialized healthcare professionals and organizations capable of helping you with your arthritis have grown in number and expertise. They all agree that people with arthritis who communicate well with their doctors and consultants stand a better chance of successfully managing their condition.

Understanding arthritis

Arthritis is not a single condition but a variety of many different conditions that can affect the joints at any stage of life, from the early days of childhood until the closing stages of old age. Arthritis has two key characteristics – joint pain and inflammation. Some people with arthritis have only pain but most have a combination of the two. To make sense of arthritis it is important to understand some key general information, such as the types of joint and the causes and consequences of joint inflammation.

Anyone can develop arthritis. It affects men and women of all ages, and sometimes even children.

The characteristics of arthritis

The hallmark of arthritis is joint inflammation, which leads to tenderness and swelling. People with arthritis usually complain of joint stiffness, too.

The many types of arthritis can be divided into three main groups: inflammatory, non-inflammatory, and connective tissue arthritis.

In inflammatory arthritis, there is swelling of the soft tissues around a joint. Stiffness is most marked in the morning, when it may last an hour or more. Inflammatory arthritis may be acute (short term),

such as gout, or chronic (long term), such as rheumatoid arthritis.

Non-inflammatory forms of arthritis include torn ligaments and osteoarthritis. In the latter, there is more bony swelling and less soft-tissue swelling than in inflammatory arthritis and stiffness usually occurs at rest or after exercise.

The third group consists of inflammatory conditions, such as lupus and fibromyalgia, that affect the connective tissues.

When only one joint is involved the condition is sometimes called a monoarthritis. When many joints are affected the condition may be described as a polyarthritis.

Q&A

Are women usually more affected by arthritis than men?

Yes. It is mainly due to the fact that impaired immunity is a significant factor. Most medical conditions in which there is impaired immunity are three times more common in women. However, other diseases, such as ankylosing spondylitis and gout, are more common in men.

Which joints are affected?

Most forms of arthritis affect the small joints in the hands and feet, and the large joints of the knees and hips, although any joint can be involved.

Different forms of arthritis affect different joints. Osteoarthritis, for example, usually affects the top two joints of the fingers and the base of the thumb, as well as the knees and the hips. Rheumatoid arthritis usually involves the bottom two joints of the fingers and thumbs, and also the wrists. Gout characteristically affects the joint at the base of the big toe.

Challenges to overcome

People with arthritis often have to face difficulties and challenges that can compromise their way of life, although many of them can also be overcome.

There are four main reasons for these challenges. First, the pain and inflammation immediately limit what you can do. Second,

the progressive damage to your joints makes your muscles weak, making you less active. Third, the chronic pain wears you out and restricts the amount of exercise you are able to do. Finally, your treatment, as well as related and associated conditions, can put a strain on your quality of life.

Many forms of arthritis, particularly rheumatoid arthritis, are associated with changes in the skin or internal organs because they affect all the systems in the body, not just locally in the joints.

Who is affected by arthritis?

Anyone can develop arthritis. It affects men and women of all ages, and sometimes even children (see p.182). No-one knows for sure

A COMMON CONDITION
Arthritis is a common condition in countries throughout the world and characteristically affects people in later life.

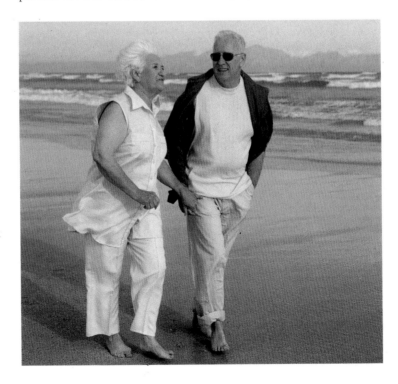

TYPES OF JOINT

Joints are the sites in the body where two bones make contact. Most joints have a space called the synovial cavity between the two bones. These synovial joints, such as the hip and elbow, allow movement and provide mechanical support.

Some joints, such as the joints of the spine, are connected by discs of cartilage and permit some movement; others, such as the bones of the skull, are bound by fibrous tissue and permit no movement at all. In general, the joints that allow movement are the joints involved in arthritis.

Although they are different, synovial joints share one underlying similarity: the surfaces of the two bones, where they meet, are covered in a thin superficial layer of cartilage called the synovial membrane. Deeper layers of cartilage are able to absorb shocks.

Synovial joints move in various ways. Some, such as the wrist, have a wide range of movement but do not move far in any direction. Hinge joints, such as the elbow, allow plenty of movement but only in a single plane. Ball-and-socket joints, such as the hip, have a wide range of movement in several directions.

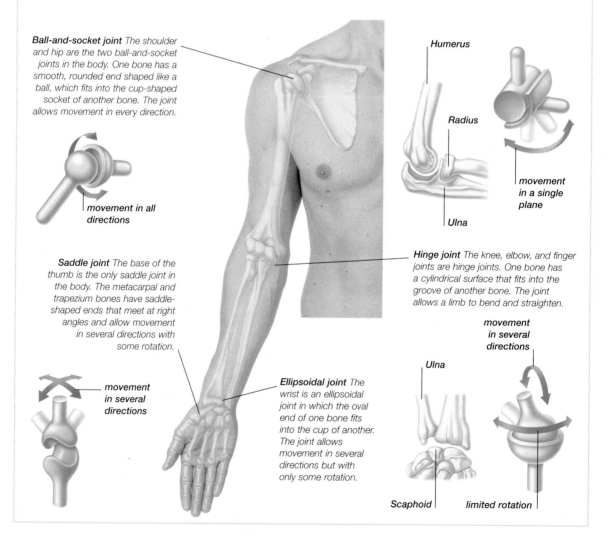

Ball-and-socket joint *The shoulder and hip are the two ball-and-socket joints in the body. One bone has a smooth, rounded end shaped like a ball, which fits into the cup-shaped socket of another bone. The joint allows movement in every direction.*

movement in all directions

Saddle joint *The base of the thumb is the only saddle joint in the body. The metacarpal and trapezium bones have saddle-shaped ends that meet at right angles and allow movement in several directions with some rotation.*

movement in several directions

Ellipsoidal joint *The wrist is an ellipsoidal joint in which the oval end of one bone fits into the cup of another. The joint allows movement in several directions but with only some rotation.*

Humerus

Radius

Ulna

movement in a single plane

Hinge joint *The knee, elbow, and finger joints are hinge joints. One bone has a cylindrical surface that fits into the groove of another bone. The joint allows a limb to bend and straighten.*

movement in several directions

Ulna

Scaphoid

limited rotation

why some people develop arthritis and not others, but there is a great deal of information about who is most at risk.

Depending on a range of genetic and environmental factors, you might be more likely than others to develop a particular type of arthritis. These risk factors vary between diseases and also differ between ages, sexes, and ethnic groups. (See individual types of arthritis for more information.)

Arthritis usually affects people in later life, although this is not as straightforward as it sounds for two reasons. First, the start of arthritis, especially osteoarthritis, occurs mainly in old age. Second, the arthritis that people develop at a younger age has a cumulative and longstanding effect over time.

What is inflammation?

The process of inflammation is the first response that our immune systems take to combat infection or to remove irritation. The response is essential to our survival as it helps us to protect ourselves and deal with a wide range of unwanted risks, such as disease-causing bacteria. In the usual course of events, the inflammation dies down and the affected tissues return to normal.

Classically, inflammation has a quintet of features – redness, heat, swelling, pain, and loss of

function. In arthritis, only swelling and pain are present to any great extent, with loss of function being an inevitable consequence.

Redness and heat are caused by an increased blood supply to a particular part of the body, such as a joint. Blood vessels upstream of the joint become wider, while those downstream are narrowed. These changes cause the inflamed joint to swell. White blood cells accumulate and release a variety of active materials into the inflamed joint. The combination of the tissue swelling and the active substances from the white cells cause the joint to be painful.

THE HEALTHY JOINT

The cartilage and synovial fluid play an important role in the health of a joint. The cartilage protecting the ends of the bones has to be smooth, springy, and tough. The fluid provides the nutrients the cartilage needs to renew itself and filters out the debris as the surface layers of cartilage are worn away. The movement of the joint constantly presses and releases the cartilage like a sponge, allowing nourishment to reach the deeper layers of cartilage and waste to be removed.

SYNOVIAL JOINT
This cutaway shows the principal features of every synovial (freely movable) joint.

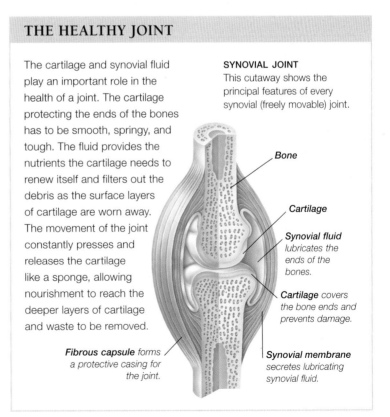

Bone

Cartilage

Synovial fluid lubricates the ends of the bones.

Cartilage covers the bone ends and prevents damage.

Fibrous capsule *forms a protective casing for the joint.*

Synovial membrane secretes lubricating synovial fluid.

The main types of arthritis

Arthritis is very common, with 200 identifiable types. Only a few, however, such as osteoarthritis and rheumatoid arthritis, affect people in significant numbers. Arthritis develops in various settings and for a number of reasons: wear and tear of the bones in a joint; longstanding (chronic) inflammation of the soft tissues around a joint; genetic predisposition; the accumulation of crystals in a joint; and an infection in a joint. As a result, many conditions are categorized under the term arthritis.

Trauma or a major injury or operation on a joint may lead to osteoarthritis at that site later in life.

Osteoarthritis

Osteoarthritis is the most common form of arthritis. It is usually considered to be a degenerative "wear-and-tear" condition that is associated with aging, although younger people can also develop it following an injury.

If you have osteoarthritis you will probably find that only one joint, or a small number of joints, are affected. The most likely are the top joints of your fingers, the base joint of your thumb, your hips, or your knees.

Osteoarthritis is more common in the knee than in the hip; taken together, the hips and knees are affected in 10–20 per cent of people aged over 65 and are a major cause of pain and disability in elderly people.

About 8.5 million people in the UK have osteoarthritis, but only a million actively seek treatment. The others never realize they have it, nor suffer any pain, although it may be seen when people are X-rayed for other reasons.

Risk factors

Usually, several risk factors need to be present before osteoarthritis develops. The main factors include age, gender, obesity, occupation,

Q&A

Can changes in the weather make my osteoarthritis worse?

Cold wet weather may make your joints feel worse but there is no strong evidence to suggest that your osteoarthritis is affected. People often think that if they moved to a warm dry climate their arthritis would improve. However, osteoarthritis is just as common in warmer regions as in colder climates.

SITES OF ARTHRITIS

Osteoarthritis (opposite) and rheumatoid arthritis (see p.18) tend to affect certain joints, although any joint might be involved. The main joints affected by osteoarthritis are the hips, knees, hands, and feet. Rheumatoid arthritis targets a wider range of joints and varies considerably from one person to another. The hands and feet are often involved, as are the wrists, ankles, shoulders, and knees. Less commonly affected are the elbows, jaws, and bones in the neck and lower back.

SKELETON
- Osteoarthritis
- Rheumatoid arthritis

Jaw
Neck
Sternoclavicular joint
Shoulder
Elbow
Lower back
Hip
Knee
Ankle
Foot
Toes

Base of thumb
Wrist

JOINTS OF THE HAND
Osteoarthritis may affect the top and middle joints of the fingers and the base of the thumb. Rheumatoid arthritis may affect the knuckles and the middle joints of the fingers, as well as the wrist.

genetics, trauma, or any previous inflammation of a joint.

■ **AGE** The dominant risk factor of osteoarthritis is age. It usually starts after age 45 and rises steeply with increasing age. Most people aged over 65 years have some evidence of osteoarthritis. As more people live longer, osteoarthritis will become more common, probably because they will experience increasing muscle weakness and they will be less able to repair worn or damaged tissues.

■ **GENDER** For most joints, esepcially those in the knees and the hands, osteoarthritis is more common – and also more severe – in women than in men.

■ **OBESITY** Those people who are more than 25 per cent above their target healthy weight are markedly more at risk of osteoarthritis. This is most likely because of pressure of the increased weight on the joints. The knee is at particular risk. At the same time, people who are overweight or obese increase their chances of osteoarthritis worsening once it has developed.

■ **TRAUMA** A major injury to, or operation on, a joint may lead to osteoarthritis at that site later in life. If you do a hard and repetitive activity you may injure a joint and

RUNNING IN THE FAMILY
Nodal osteoarthritis is a condition that may be inherited, particularly on the female side of the family.

In osteoarthritis the surface of the cartilage breaks down and wears away so that the bones under the cartilage start to rub together.

make it prone to osteoarthritis. If you exercise too soon after a joint injury has had time to heal properly, the joint may also develop osteoarthritis.

Occupations such as farming make osteoarthritis of the hip more likely; footballers are prone to osteoarthritis of the knee. Occupations involving knee bending, squatting, and heavy lifting are associated with osteoarthritis of the knee.

■ **GENETICS** The presence of certain genes plays a role in the common form of nodal osteoarthritis (see p.18), which particularly affects the hands of middle-aged women. In osteoarthritis of the knee and hip, heredity plays a smaller, though still significant, role. General osteoarthritis probably has a genetic basis, too.

Genes that are likely to be involved in the common forms of osteoarthritis include the vitamin D receptor gene, the insulin-like growth factor genes, the cartilage

oligomeric protein genes and the HLA region (see p.200). There are some very rare but dramatic forms of osteoarthritis that start at a young age and run in families. These are linked with single genes that affect the protein collagen, which is an essential component of healthy cartilage.

What happens?

Osteoarthritis often develops slowly and varies from person to person: some people have only minor symptoms, but in others the condition can be very severe.

The primary site is the cartilage that covers the ends of the bones in a joint. Healthy cartilage lets bones glide over one another and absorbs the energy from movement. In osteoarthritis, the surface of the cartilage breaks down and wears away so that the bones under the cartilage start to rub together. The results are pain, swelling, and reduced movement.

Q&A

Last winter I injured my knee while I was skiing – does this mean I may develop osteoarthritis later in life?

Yes, it's possible, particularly if you damaged the cartilage. In addition, if you didn't wait for the injury to heal completely before you returned to physical exercise, you may have made it more likely that the joint is affected by osteoarthritis – but no-one can say when.

The swelling is usually the result of lumps forming on the bone but sometimes it can be due to increased fluid in the joint. In some cases, the joint makes an abnormal noise, or crepitus, when it moves. Affected joints often stiffen after exercise, sometimes known as "gelling". Some people with osteoarthritis feel stiff in the morning, but this lasts only a few minutes. Osteoarthritis does not affect internal organs.

Eventually, the affected joint loses its normal shape and becomes deformed. Small spurs called osteophytes often form at the end of the bones. Small pieces of cartilage or bone may break off and float inside the joint space, causing further pain and damage. In some ways osteoarthritis represents joint failure, which can be minimal or complete, depending on its severity.

Osteoarthritis of the knee

When osteoarthritis affects the knee, particularly among people between their late 50s and early 70s, it can be very complicated. Osteoarthritis of the knee is more common in women than men and generally affects both knees.

You may have more chance of developing osteoarthritis of the knee if you are overweight, have osteoarthritis in another joint, or have had a previous sporting injury or knee surgery, in particular cartilage removal.

Often, however, there is no obvious cause. Pain is usually felt at the front and sides of the knee. In the later stages, the knees can become bent and deformed.

Osteoarthritis of the hip

Women and men are equally affected by osteoarthritis of the hip. It can start in their 40s but

OSTEOARTHRITIS OF THE HIP

Mechanical wear and tear can cause the cartilage of the hip joint to deteriorate and unprotected bone to be exposed. As a result, the space between the head of the thigh bone and the socket of the pelvis narrows to the point where the two bones touch. Prolonged contact and damage leads to the development of bony spurs, or osteophytes. The hip becomes painful and restricted in its movements. Painkillers may bring some relief but serious cases will require surgery to replace the hip (see p.92).

OSTEOARTHRITIC HIP
This X-ray of an osteoarthritic hip joint shows narrowing of the space between the head of the thigh bone and the socket in the pelvis.

Osteophytes (bony growths) form on the socket of the pelvis.

Cartilage normally protects bone underneath.

Joint capsule becomes inflamed.

Exposed bone

JOINT CAPSULE OF AN OSTEOARTHRITIC HIP

more usually later in life. One or both hips are equally likely to be involved. Certain hip problems that were present at birth or have developed in childhood may later lead to osteoarthritis. Some people have anatomical features that predispose them to osteoarthritis. For example, in certain cases, the acetabulum – the cup of the pelvic socket into which the head of the thigh bone sits – is not as well developed as it should be.

Hip pain from osteoarthritis is usually at the front of the groin, but it can also occur in the buttock or in the knee, when it is considered to be "referred" pain.

Osteoarthritis of the hands

This condition mainly involves women and commonly starts in the late 40s or early 50s, often around the time of the menopause (see p.192). It chiefly affects the joint at the base of the thumb, and the joints at the top of the fingers. Although the fingers become knobbly and sometimes slightly bent, they work well and rarely cause long-term problems.

Nodal osteoarthritis affects the finger joints. These joints are swollen and tender, especially at the beginning, and then develop firm, bony, knobbly swellings. When these affect the top joints of the fingers they are called Heberden's nodes, after the 18th-century British physician who first described them.

In some cases, similar bony swellings – called Bouchard's nodes after the 19th-century French pathologist – appear on the joints in the middle of the fingers. By the time these two types of node have formed, the joints are relatively free from pain and tenderness.

People with nodal osteoarthritis in middle age are more likely to develop osteoarthritis of the knee during old age.

Rheumatoid arthritis

Around 400,000 adults in the UK have rheumatoid arthritis, making it the commonest form of inflammatory arthritis. Although its cause is unknown, it is usually thought to be an autoimmune disease in which the body starts to attack itself – but the evidence for this is incomplete.

Rheumatoid arthritis can occur at any age, but it is more common in later life. Usually, many joints are involved (see p.15). It is a long-term (chronic) disease that is characterized by persistent joint inflammation. This, over a prolonged period of time, results in irreversible joint damage.

Risk factors

Gender, genetics, and age are the most important risk factors for rheumatoid arthritis. Others include heavy smoking, obesity, a history of blood transfusions, and a shorter fertile period in women associated with low levels of reproductive hormones. Drinking coffee and trauma have been suggested as risk factors, but the evidence is very inconclusive.

■ **GENDER** A dominant risk factor is geneder – up to three-quarters of people with rheumatoid arthritis are women. Research suggests that in a population of 100,000 adults there will be approximately 36 new cases of rheumatoid arthritis in women and 14 in men per year in the UK. The incidence rate rises steeply as people grow older, especially in men.

■ **GENETICS** Genes play a significant role in the development of rheumatoid arthritis. Up to 60 per cent of the predisposition to rheumatoid arthritis is explained by genetic factors (see p.200). The condition is strongly related to the presence of a protein on the surface of white blood cells (leucocytes) called HLA–DR4. Most evidence suggests that genetics contribute mainly to the severity of the disease rather than to disease susceptibility.

■ **AGE** Rheumatoid arthritis can begin at any age. It was viewed traditionally as starting in young adulthood, with a peak age of

RHEUMATOID ARTHRITIS OF THE HANDS

Rheumatoid arthritis usually affects a number of joints, often the same joints similarly – but not always simultaneously – on both sides of the body. Although the joints affected vary from person to person, several specific joints are more commonly involved than others. In the hand, these include the base of the thumb, the middle joints of the fingers, the knuckles, and the wrists.

As the rheumatoid arthritis develops, the cartilage is damaged, and the joints swell and become inflamed, causing pain and restricted movement. Moving the hand may cause a creaking sound called crepitus. Eventually, the fingers bend away from the thumb.

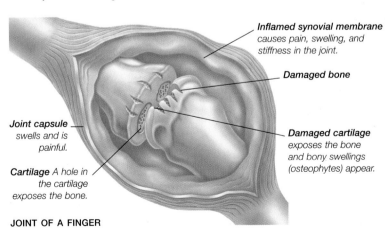

Inflamed synovial membrane causes pain, swelling, and stiffness in the joint.

Damaged bone

Joint capsule swells and is painful.

Damaged cartilage exposes the bone and bony swellings (osteophytes) appear.

Cartilage A hole in the cartilage exposes the bone.

JOINT OF A FINGER

HAND AFFECTED BY RHEUMATOID ARTHRITIS
This X-ray of a hand with severe rheumatoid arthritis shows the swollen and inflamed joints (orange) that are a feature of the condition. As the cartilage deteriorates, the bones become damaged.

onset between 20 and 45 years. For unknown reasons, this has changed and the average age of onset has increased to 60 years.

What happens?

The synovial membrane of one or more joints becomes inflamed, causing pain, swelling, and stiffness. In the early stages, the swelling involves only soft tissue and there may be an increase of fluid in the joint (an effusion).

Stiffness is characteristic of any type of inflammatory arthritis and is usually present in the morning – it can last for an hour or two, but in severe cases can persist all day. The inflammation spreads to the synovial sheaths that protect and lubricate the tendons linking the bones of the joints to the muscles that move them.

As the disease progresses, the inflammation persists for some unknown reason and results in progressive and usually irreversible damage to joints. The more the inflammation, the greater the risks of damage. Bony swellings appear and deformity develops as the joints become damaged and begin to fail. The muscles weaken, partly through lack of use and partly from the effects of a generalized inflammatory condition.

Rheumatoid arthritis starts in different ways. Usually, it starts slowly, with intermittent pain and swelling in some joints, especially in the fingers, wrists, and feet. The

symptoms gradually worsen until it is self-evident to the individual that there is something wrong with the joints. In perhaps 20 per cent of cases, the disease starts very suddenly: one day the individual is normal and the next many joints are painful, swollen, and stiff.

In some people the disease starts in less usual ways. For example, it may involve a single joint. In others, the disease comes and goes repeatedly, often over several years, before becoming persistent. Occasionally, it starts with pain and stiffness around the shoulders and so mimics a condition called polymyalgic rheumatism.

The way the disease progresses is very variable. Some people have a mild disease with few problems and can live normal lives. For others, the disease may enter a period of sustained remission, without returning, or else follows an intermittent course, when flare-ups are followed by remissions that do not last long.

Many people have chronic persistent arthritis, in which continuing disease activity has added flare-ups from time to time. Although highly unusual, a few people have a persisting severe disease that remains active despite the best efforts of most therapies.

Disability

Taken together, inflammation and damage to joints cause marked disability. This varies with time and is unique to an individual, depending on the exact ways the joints are involved. Some people with rheumatoid arthritis are simply unable to do normal things. The disability is also psychological and social. For example, many, though by no means all, people with rheumatoid arthritis find it difficult to work and some will need to leave their job as a result. (See Day-to-day Living, p.134.)

Ankylosing spondylitis

This inflammatory disease affects the spine predominantly and can result in marked stiffness or even fusion of the spine (see Stiffening of the Spine, right). "Ankylosing" is another word for stiffening, while "spondylitis" means inflammation of the spine.

The cause of ankylosing spondylitis is unknown. Unlike rheumatoid arthritis the disorder is not associated with the presence of rheumatoid factor in the blood (see p.41); nor does it show any features of autoimmunity. The two sacroiliac joints, which connect the spine to the pelvis and do not have a synovium, are also involved.

Around 200,000 UK adults have the disorder. Some studies put this figure at 1 in 1,000 adults, whilst others suggest that a mild version of ankylosing spondylitis affects up to 1 per cent of adults.

Risk factors

Genetics and gender are the main risk factors. It is sometimes related to infection so some experts think there may be an infectious trigger.

■ **GENETICS** A gene called HLA-B27 plays a role in the condition. Up to 95 per cent of those with the ankylosing spondylitis have the gene, compared to under 10 per cent of the general population.

STIFFENING OF THE SPINE

In ankylosing spondylitis, the joints between the vertebrae of the spine become inflamed, starting at the sacroiliac joints where the spine links with the pelvis. The ligaments around the joints accumulate calcium salts and become hard. New bone forms once the inflammation subsides. As a result, the spine stiffens and becomes inflexible. Eventually, in severe cases, the joints may fuse and prevent movement. The joints connecting the vertebrae to the ribs may become inflamed, which often makes breathing difficult.

X–RAY OF THE SPINE
This X–ray of the lumbar region of a spine affected with ankylosing spondylitis shows severe deformity of the vertebrae, with the rounded spine curving outwards.

Vertebra becomes deformed and fixed in position.

Disc cartilage becomes inflexible.

Ligaments accumulate calcium salts and become hard.

CROSS SECTION (SIDE VIEW) OF SPINE

■ **GENDER** Men are most often affected by ankylosing spondylitis, particularly those in their 20s and 30s. The ratio of men to women with ankylosing spondylitis is about 5 to 1. When the disease affects women it tends to be milder than in men.

What happens?

The initial features of ankylosing spondylitis are stiffness, an ache in the lower back, and reduced movement of the spine. The stiffness is present in the morning and often lasts for several hours.

Some people with ankylosing spondylitis have only mild aches and pains that progress slowly over months or years. Others have a more active disease that leads to feelings of ill-health and fatigue, and to potential loss of weight.

In addition, the disorder is associated with iritis, which causes an acutely inflamed red eye and requires immediate medical attention to avoid permanent damage to the eye.

Over time, the disease may clear up or cause only minor stiffness; or it may become more serious as the stiffness progresses, with limited movement of the spine that results in a hunched posture, rounded spine, and a flat chest. Arthritis of other joints, such as the knee or hip, usually resolves with time. Only a very few patients develop a progressive destructive arthritis of their joints.

Psoriatic arthritis

Psoriatic arthritis is not a common disorder – around 100,000 adults in the UK are affected. It is an inflammatory arthritis associated with the skin condition psoriasis, although this is not inevitable and, in most instances, is not usually a consequence. In fact, sometimes the arthritis develops first. About 1 in 50 people has psoriasis; of these, about 1 in 14 develops psoriatic arthritis.

Psoriatic arthritis affects men and women in equal measure and usually starts in middle age. The cause is unknown, although genetics probably play a small part. Like ankylosing spondylitis, it may be triggered by an infection.

What happens?

Many people with psoriatic arthritis experience inflammation in one or two joints, such as a knee or ankle. In other people, it involves the top joint of the fingers (see left). Sometimes, many joints are affected and the disease is similar to rheumatoid arthritis.

About a third of people with psoriatic arthritis also have spinal disease, with back or neck pain due to spinal inflammation. Tendons and the site where tendons are attached to bones may also become inflamed. This can cause pain in the Achilles tendon, in the heels, and around the top of the thigh bone.

Gout

Gout is a condition with a clearly identified cause – the presence of uric acid crystals in the synovial fluid of a joint. Gout affects the joints, particularly the big toe, where it can be very painful. In fact, during an acute attack, this condition can be the most painful arthritis of all.

Gout is a disorder of uric acid metabolism. It affects between 1 and 2 per cent of UK adults and usually develops in middle age. Gout is usually preceded by a period of high uric acid levels in the blood. It is generally related to various lifestyle factors, such as eating red meat and drinking alcohol excessively.

Risk factors

Genetics and gender are the main risk factors. The frequency of gout increases with age. Some of the uric acid that contributes to gout comes from a high intake of purines, essential molecules found in lentils, dried beans, sardines, shellfish, and organ meats. Most of the uric acid comes from within the body when purines and proteins are broken down.

■ **GENETICS** Many people with gout have an inherited tendency for their uric acid levels to be high.

■ **GENDER** Gout is about three times more common in men than in women. Gout rarely affects women before they reach the menopause.

Q&A

Does everyone with high uric acid levels have gout?

No. And curiously, many patients who experience an acute attack of gout do not have raised uric acid levels. Nevertheless, it is true to say that the higher the uric acid levels, the more likely the chance of an attack of gout.

■ **MEDICAL TREATMENT** Uric acid levels may increase after medical treatment. Cancer treatment causes cells to be broken down and purines to be released from DNA. Thiazide diuretics, such as bendrofluazide, for high blood pressure also raise uric acid levels.

What happens?

Gout can be triggered by illness, surgery, trauma, or a metabolic disturbance. Acute gout causes agony. There is a sudden onset of pain in a single joint which is hot, red, and very tender to the touch. Some people have recurrent episodes; in others, gout is like rheumatoid arthritis, becoming chronic and destructive.

Uric acid is normally excreted in urine. When the balance between the amount produced and the amount excreted is upset, blood levels rise. When these are too high, crystals form and collect in the white cells in joints and other tissues. This can cause an acute arthritis with intense local pain.

Gout affects the joints, particularly the big toe, where it can be very painful. In fact, during an acute attack, this condition can be the most painful arthritis of all.

In gout, high levels of uric acid in the blood cause crystals of uric acid to accumulate in the synovial fluid and joint capsule of one or more joints. In an attack of gout, which may come without warning, the pain can be unbearable. The affected joint turns red with inflammation and swells up.

Gout most commonly and traditionally targets the joint at the base of the big toe where the pain is also the most excruciating. Others joints that can be affected include the elbows, knees, ankles, wrists, and hands.

The sharp, needle-like crystals also accumulate in other parts of the body – for example, under the skin where the white deposits are known as tophi. These tophi are conventionally looked for on the earlobes, but they can occur at many sites, including the soft tissues of the hands and feet. Crystals may also accumulate in the kidneys where they form stones and can cause renal failure.

In some people, the symptoms of pseudogout are very similar to those in rheumatoid arthritis and osteoarthritis.

Pseudogout

Like gout, acute arthritis can be caused when crystals of calcium pyrophosphate dihydrate are deposited in joints, particularly the knee and less often the big toe. This is known as pseudogout because of its similarity to gout.

Pseudogout affects more men than women when compared with gout, but it usually occurs later in life. It may also run in families. In some people, the symptoms of pseudogout are very similar to those in rheumatoid arthritis and osteoarthritis.

The exact source of the crystals and why they cause acute arthritis are unknown. There may be a link with abnormal connective tissue or cartilage, or with other disorders, such as an underactive thyroid gland, excess iron storage, an overactive parathyroid gland, and other causes of excess calcium in the blood. Episodes of pseudogout can follow surgery, metabolic disturbances, or an injury to a joint.

Crystals may collect in the cartilage around joints, especially in elderly people, without causing symptoms. Many elderly people with osteoarthritis can develop pseudogout when the crystals interact with their condition.

Q&A

Can tuberculosis cause arthritis?

Yes. Chronic infections such as tuberculosis can cause arthritis. About 1 per cent of people with tuberculosis develop an associated arthritis. It particularly involves the spine, hips, knees, wrists, or ankles. It often starts slowly and usually involves just one joint. Symptoms include a low-grade fever, increased sweating, fever at night, reduced joint mobility, and some swelling and tenderness of the joints.

Arthritis and infection

Many important but relatively uncommon forms of arthritis are due to infections with viruses, bacteria, or fungi. They can occur by themselves or sometimes, in the case of infective arthritis due to bacteria, can complicate a pre-existing inflammatory arthritis. They vary in their appearance and in the course they take.

Many forms of viral illness can cause an arthritis. This is usually of minor relevance, and aches and pains occur against a background of feeling generally unwell. A viral arthritis tends to affect many joints and involves joint pain rather than inflammation, with characteristic pain and stiffness. It often occurs in the later stages of a viral illness and may come with a mild fever. Medical attention is needed to prevent the joint from becoming permanently stiff.

Acute bacterial infection tends to cause arthritis in one or more joints, which become hot, swollen, and red. There is usually a fever, too. Rarely, a sudden septic arthritis can affect a joint, with a high fever and severe ill-health. People with a pre-existing arthritis are more likely to develop it.

Reactive arthritis

This inflammatory arthritis develops after a bacterial infection. It can be accompanied by rashes on the hands or feet, diarrhoea, conjunctivitis, mouth ulcers, and inflammation of the genital tract, which produces a discharge from the vagina or penis.

Reactive arthritis usually lasts for 6 months or less and rarely has any long-term consequences. About 1 per cent of people with an episode of infective diarrhoea or a sexually acquired infection develop reactive arthritis.

Lyme disease

This disease was first identified in people from Old Lyme in the US, but it is very uncommon in Europe. Initial symptoms of Lyme disease, which is caused by a bacterium (see above), include fever, fatigue, muscle pain, and a rash. After some months, over half of infected people may develop arthritis, mainly in the large joints, especially the knees.

BORRELIA BURGDORFERI
The bacterium *Borrelia burgdorferi* (coloured yellow above) causes Lyme disease in humans and is transmitted through a bite from an infected tick.

Related conditions

Many conditions involving joint pain or inflammation of soft tissues and other areas of the body may be related to arthritis. Other disorders, such as vasculitis and carpal tunnel syndrome, may accompany the different types of arthritis. If you have arthritis, you may be at a slightly increased risk of developing such disorders, but they are not an inevitable progression; any of them can also affect people who do not have arthritis, and some are rare. You should always consult your doctor to obtain the correct diagnosis and treatment if you experience any of the symptoms described here.

Lupus has no cure but drugs can do much to relieve the symptoms and control the progression of the disease.

Lupus (SLE)

Systemic lupus erythematosus (SLE), or lupus for short, is a disease that causes inflammation in many parts of the body. The areas affected may include the joints, skin, and the tissues of the lungs, heart, and kidneys. The nervous system is sometimes involved, too. However, lupus rarely causes joint damage.

Lupus is a disorder of the immune system. It is not known what triggers the disease but viral infections, stress, and hormone imbalances may be involved. Certain drugs can occasionally cause side-effects that resemble the symptoms of lupus. The disease is far more common in women than in men and is also more likely to occur in Afro–Caribbean and Asian women. Women with lupus should consult their doctor if they are thinking of having a baby. Lupus is comparatively rare in children and does not usually develop in adults once they have reached the age of 50.

Symptoms and treatment

The first symptoms are often aches and pain in the joints, particularly in the hands and feet. Another major symptom is a red skin rash, which typically spreads across the nose and cheeks – this is called the butterfly rash. However, a red rash can appear elsewhere on the body (see below). In addition, depression and a feeling of general fatigue are common.

Some people develop persistent mouth ulcers and experience hair loss. Inflammation of the lining of the heart and lungs can cause chest pain and shortness of breath. If the kidneys are affected, serious complications may arise, such as high blood pressure and kidney failure, but these are rare.

Lupus is highly variable. Many people are affected mildly while others may have severe symptoms that intermittently flare up and then subside for long periods. Permanent improvement is very rare. Lupus has no cure but drugs (see p.87) can do much to relieve the symptoms and control the progression of the disease.

LUPUS SKIN RASH
A blotchy red rash on the skin is a common feature of lupus. The skin rashes tend to become worse if they are exposed to sunlight or ultraviolet radiation. In some instances, sunlight may even act as a trigger and cause the disease to flare up.

Fibromyalgia

The term fibromyalgia describes a collection of symptoms, the most important of which is persistent pain in many areas of the body. Fibromyalgia affects the muscles and other connective tissues, such as tendons and ligaments, and is not a joint disorder as such.

The cause of fibromyalgia is not known, but it may be linked to stress, anxiety, or depression. About 90 per cent of people with fibromyalgia are women over the age of 40. Although this disorder may persist for many months or years, it does not cause damage to muscles or joints and will not lead to the development of arthritis or make existing arthritis worse.

Symptoms and treatment

The pain may occur anywhere, often on both sides of the body at once, and is usually experienced as widespread aching and stiffness. Typically, several small sites in particular areas – such as at the base of the skull and around the shoulderblades and breastbone – are painful when pressed. Doctors use the number and distribution of these "tender points" to diagnose fibromyalgia (see p.28).

Poor posture can contribute to back pain, so you should check that you are not putting strain on soft tissues by sitting incorrectly at your desk or while driving.

Around 90 per cent of people with fibromyalgia are affected by severe fatigue and have problems with sleeping. Other associated symptoms include headaches, irregular bowel movements that alternate between diarrhoea and constipation (known as irritable bowel syndrome), and a frequent need to urinate.

Fibromyalgia can be difficult to treat, although the symptoms may be eased in various ways. For example, painkillers may bring some relief and your doctor may prescribe low-dose antidepressants to improve disturbed sleep. Self-help measures, such as low-impact exercise and applying gentle heat to painful areas, may also help.

Lower back pain

Lower back pain is one of the most common health complaints in adults. It can have many causes but is most frequently the result of a minor injury to the soft tissues of the back.

Symptoms and treatment

An acute pain in the lower back that develops suddenly is often due to a physical activity, such as lifting a heavy weight, that puts excessive strain on muscles or tendons. An injury of this type can cause a sharp pain in one specific place or a more widespread, dull aching, as well as stiffness when you bend down.

THE TENDER POINTS OF FIBROMYALGIA

Fibromyalgia can be difficult to diagnose so doctors rely on the presence of tender points, located in 9 symmetrical pairs, at particular sites around the body. Although this technique is not foolproof because tenderness can vary from day to day, fibromyalgia may be confirmed if 11 of the 18 points are tender when pressed. The pairs of tender points can be found in the following locations: at the base of the skull, at the base of the neck, on top of the shoulders, on the inside edge of the shoulderblades, below the elbows, at the top of the breastbone, at the top of the hips, at the top of the outer thighs, and on the fat pad just above the inside of the knees.

Breastbone

Knee

Base of skull

Neck

Shoulderblade

Shoulder

Elbow

Hip

Thigh

Poor posture is a more gradual way of contributing to back pain, so you should check that you are not putting strain on soft tissues by sitting incorrectly at your desk (see p.178) or while driving.

Another cause of back pain is a condition known commonly as a "slipped disc", in which one of the shock-absorbing pads of cartilage between two vertebrae is displaced (prolapsed) or damaged. If the disc presses against one of the nerves in the spine, you may experience severe pain, as well as numbness and tingling in one leg. Persistent lower back pain and sciatica are frequently related to some types of arthritis, such as osteoarthritis or ankylosing spondylitis, which affect the joints of the spine.

Back pain due to minor tissue damage usually clears up within about 2 weeks. Your doctor may suggest that you take painkillers and you could try self-help measures, such as applying a heat pad or an ice pack to your back, to ease the symptoms. Bed rest may help if you are in severe pain, but do not prolong it for more than a day or two.

Localized soft-tissue disorders

The pain and inflammation in the following common conditions is usually confined to the soft tissues around specific joints.

INCIDENCE OF BACK PAIN

Back pain seems to strike when you are least expecting it or when a relatively minor action triggers a disproportionately painful episode. Statistics show that back problems are most likely to trouble you between the ages of 30 and 50, when the discs between your vertebrae are at their most vulnerable.

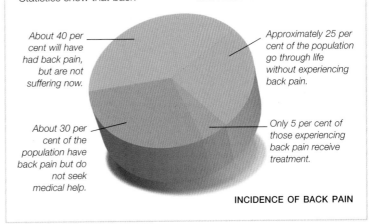

About 40 per cent will have had back pain, but are not suffering now.

Approximately 25 per cent of the population go through life without experiencing back pain.

About 30 per cent of the population have back pain but do not seek medical help.

Only 5 per cent of those experiencing back pain receive treatment.

INCIDENCE OF BACK PAIN

Bursitis

Joints are cushioned by fluid-filled sacs called bursae, which help to reduce friction. In bursitis, a bursa becomes inflamed and tender, making the joint stiff and painful to move. The most common sites of bursitis are the knee, elbow, and shoulder. Persistently repeated movement or pressure are the usual causes; more rarely, it may be caused by an infection. Inflammatory arthritis can make you more susceptible to bursitis.

Resting the joint, applying ice packs, and anti-inflammatory drugs often relieve the symptoms, which usually go away after a week. If the bursitis recurs or remains troublesome, your doctor may suggest draining the bursa.

PRACTICAL TIPS

LOWER BACK PAIN

If you suddenly have an acute attack of pain in your lower back:

● Stay calm and don't panic. Just relax and breathe deeply.

● Keep your spine straight to take the weight off the discs of cartilage in your spine. Lie down or sit, whichever is the most comfortable, and rest.

● Contact your doctor if the pain does not ease up.

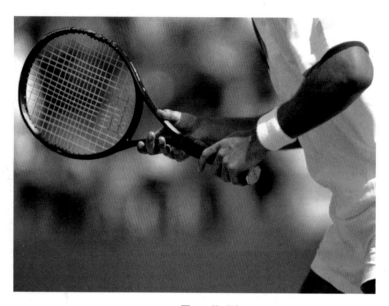

TENNIS ELBOW
This painful condition occurs when a tendon becomes inflamed and painful at the point where it is attached to a bone in the elbow. It often results from overuse or repetitive movements.

Tendinitis

Tendinitis is the inflammation of a tendon, one of the tough, flexible cords that attach muscle to bone or muscle to muscle. It is often caused by injury or overstrain and occasionally by arthritis. In rare cases, the inflammation is due to an infection. In tendinitis, the synovium (the sheath of tissue surrounding the tendon) often becomes inflamed at the same time; this accompanying disorder is known as tenosynovitis.

Tendinitis and tenosynovitis cause pain and stiffness around a joint; the area may be swollen, red, and warm to touch. Tendons in the shoulder, elbow, knee, and heel are most likely to be affected. If you have rheumatoid arthritis, you may develop tenosynovitis in your fingers. Your doctor may prescribe drugs to reduce the pain and inflammation.

Tennis elbow

This condition, in which the outer part of the elbow is inflamed and painful, is not necessarily due to playing tennis. Known medically as lateral epicondylitis, it most often occurs when strenuous repetitive movements, such as those used in heavy manual work, cause tiny tears in the tendon. The condition may also be caused by a direct blow to the arm or may be a complication of arthritis.

Symptoms include pain and tenderness around the bony point of the elbow as well as stiffness of movement. The pain is caused by damage to the tendon that attaches the muscles of the forearm to the upper arm bone (humerus). If you continue to overuse the arm, you may cause further damage to the tendon, and the pain and stiffness may gradually get worse.

For mild tennis elbow you can rest the arm, apply ice packs to the painful area, and take anti-inflammatory drugs. For more severe damage, your doctor may suggest physiotherapy, which includes gentle stretching exercises and possibly ultrasound treatment. If the condition does not improve within a few weeks, your doctor may inject a corticosteroid into your elbow joint.

Plantar fasciitis

This painful foot disorder is the inflammation of the plantar fascia on the sole of the foot. Plantar fasciitis, also called heel spur, is usually the result of an injury. Older people are prone to it because the tissues in their feet have lost some elasticity and their heels are less able to absorb shock.

The main risk factors are sudden weight gain, which can put extra strain on the feet, and existing foot problems, such as flat feet and high arches.

The pain of plantar fasciitis, which may be a severe, stabbing sensation, is felt under the bottom of the heel (see below), especially when you first stand up in the morning. Sitting down may bring temporary relief, but the pain tends to return when you stand or walk for any length of time.

Your doctor may suggest drugs that will reduce the inflammation.

Wearing an arch support in your shoe and carrying out gentle stretching exercises may also help.

Sjögren's syndrome

This condition is an immune system disorder in which the tissues of lubricating glands, especially the glands that produce tears and saliva, are inflamed. The eyes become very dry and feel gritty; a lack of saliva in the mouth often causes difficulty swallowing. In women, the glands that moisten the vagina may also be affected. Occasionally, the joints are inflamed, causing symptoms similar to those of rheumatoid arthritis. Sjögren's syndrome is far more common in women than in men, and is most likely to develop in middle age.

DRY TONGUE IN SJÖGREN'S SYNDROME
In this condition, the tongue dries out as the salivary glands start to waste away and stop producing saliva.

WHAT HAPPENS IN PLANTAR FASCIITIS

Along the sole of each foot, stretching from the heel to the ball, there is a band of tough fibrous tissue called the plantar fascia. This tissue contributes to the shape of the arch of your foot and, at the same time, gives it support. Every day, it is subject to constant stresses as you walk or run or bend your foot in any way. Plantar fasciitis occurs when an area of the plantar fascia becomes inflamed where it attaches to the calcaneus bone of the heel.

ANATOMY OF THE FOOT

Calcaneus bone of the heel

The plantar fascia (band of fibrous tissue) becomes painful and inflamed.

Metatarsal bone

Without treatment, carpal tunnel syndrome may eventually lead to permanent numbness in the hand, wasting of muscles and a weakened grip.

There is no cure for the condition but symptoms can be relieved with treatments such as artificial tears for dry eyes and, in severe cases, drugs to reduce inflammation.

Scleroderma

In scleroderma (the term means "hard skin"), the connective tissues that support and join together the various parts of the body become hardened and thick. The disease, which is believed to be an abnormality of the immune system, most commonly affects the skin and joints, although internal organs may also be damaged.

Early symptoms include Raynaud's phenomenon, in which the fingers become cold, white, and swollen. Finger joints may be stiff and painful to move. Thickening of the skin sometimes develops over wide areas of the body and the skin may feel tight.

Widespread scleroderma often affects the oesophagus (the tube that conveys food from the mouth to the stomach), stiffening the tissues, and causing difficulty with swallowing as well as digestive problems. In severe cases, the tissue damage spreads to the lungs, heart, and kidneys, impairing their function and causing long-term complications.

Scleroderma cannot be cured although treatment with drugs can slow down its progression.

Accompanying conditions

A number of potentially serious conditions, such as carpal tunnel syndrome, polymyositis, vasculitis, and osteoporosis, may accompany some of the types of arthritis. However, this link with arthritis is not inevitable. At the same time, people who do not have arthritis may develop the conditions.

Carpal tunnel syndrome

In this condition, the main nerve to the hand is compressed as it passes through the wrist, causing numbness and tingling in the hand (see p.33). Pain may be felt in the wrist and up the forearm, too.

The cause of carpal tunnel syndrome is not always obvious, but it is sometimes linked to repetitive hand movements that cause swelling of the soft tissues

REPETITIVE STRAIN
People who spend hours in front of a computer put the joints of their wrists and fingers under repeated strain and may develop carpal tunnel syndrome.

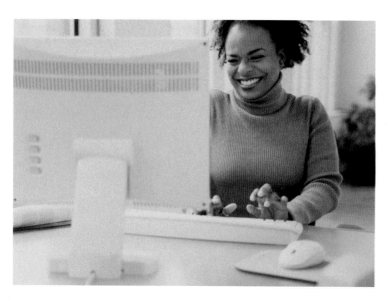

within the carpal tunnel (see right). This is why carpal tunnel syndrome is a form of repetitive strain injury. Damage to the joints of the wrist, due to injury or arthritis, may also cause narrowing of the carpal tunnel.

Many people find that their symptoms are often most severe at night or when they wake in the morning. Without treatment, carpal tunnel syndrome may eventually lead to permanent numbness in the hand, wasting of muscles and a weakened grip.

Wearing a wrist splint or practising a yoga pose called namaste (see right) may bring relief. If symptoms are particularly bad, your doctor may prescribe anti-inflammatory drugs. In some cases, surgery may relieve pressure on the median nerve.

Polymyositis and dermatomyositis

These two rare disorders are types of soft-tissue inflammation that may develop at the same time.

In polymyositis, the muscles are affected, especially around the pelvis and in the shoulders, causing weakness and pain. You may have difficulty raising your hands above your head, getting up from a chair, or climbing stairs. If the condition worsens, the muscles of the throat, chest, and heart may also be damaged, causing difficulty swallowing and shortness of breath.

CARPAL TUNNEL SYNDROME

The carpal tunnel is the gap between the wrist bones (carpals). The median nerve passes through the tunnel, underneath a band of ligament, and branches into nerves that serve the fingers and the thumb. These nerves control some of the muscles of the hand. In carpal tunnel syndrome, pressure on the median nerve causes numbness and tingling, particularly in the first and middle fingers and the thumb.

NAMASTE YOGA POSE
A yoga pose called namaste can bring relief to the pain of carpal tunnel syndrome. The palms are held together in front of the chest, with the elbows pointing out to the sides.

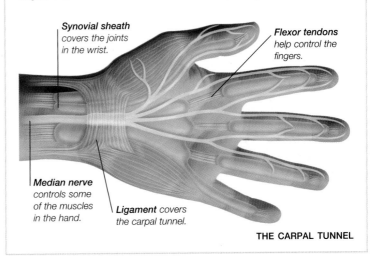

Synovial sheath covers the joints in the wrist.

Flexor tendons help control the fingers.

Median nerve controls some of the muscles in the hand.

Ligament covers the carpal tunnel.

THE CARPAL TUNNEL

In dermatomyositis, a rash occurs, most often appearing on the face and the backs of the hands. Typically, the eyelids become swollen and turn a reddish-purple. In children, severe dermatomyositis may also cause skin ulcers.

There is no cure for polymyositis and dermatomyositis, but your doctor may prescribe drug treatment to reduce inflammation and improve the symptoms.

VASCULITIS

Inflammation of the body's blood vessels, known by the general term of vasculitis, may accompany inflammatory arthritis. One form of vasculitis is giant cell arteritis (also called Horton's disease), which is caused by a response of the immune system. Giant cell arteritis usually affects the cranial and temporal arteries of the head in the elderly, causing headaches.

GIANT CELL ARTERITIS
The most characteristic feature of the condition is the presence of giant cells – one such cell can be seen at the centre of this light micrograph.

However, in the majority of children who are affected, the disorders usually disappear completely within about two years. On the other hand, adults who are affected are likely to need long-term treatment.

Polymyalgia rheumatica

In this disorder, pain and stiffness affect many muscles, mainly in the neck, shoulders, and around the hips and thighs. The symptoms, which may develop gradually but can also sometimes appear very rapidly, may include fever, night sweats, depression, and general fatigue and weakness. In some people, polymyalgia rheumatica is associated with giant cell arteritis (see left and below).

The cause of the disorder is not known. Women are more likely to be affected than men and the disorder is rare in people under the age of 50. Treatment is usually with drugs to relieve pain and reduce inflammation.

Blood vessel disorders

Inflammation of the blood vessels, known as vasculitis, sometimes occurs in conjunction with other inflammatory disorders, such as rheumatoid arthritis, although the condition can also develop in people with no previous health problems. Vasculitis can affect all types of blood vessels: arteries, veins, and capillaries. Two forms of vasculitis are described below.

■ **WEGENER'S GRANULOMATOSIS** The typical symptom of this disorder is inflammation of the blood vessels that supply the tissues of the nasal passages, lungs, and kidneys. As the disease progresses, it causes the formation of abnormal groups of cells called granulomas, which eventually replace healthy tissues.

Symptoms often first appear in the respiratory tract and can include nosebleeds, inflamed sinuses, coughing up of phlegm that is sometimes bloodstained, and shortness of breath.

These symptoms may be accompanied by fever, aches and pains, and tiredness. Sometimes the middle ear is also inflamed. If the condition affects the kidneys it may prevent the normal filtering of waste products from the blood. Long-term treatment with drugs may be needed to prevent complications arising.

■ **GIANT CELL ARTERITIS** Also known as temporal arteritis, this affects the arteries in the head and neck – most commonly the temporal arteries, which lie just beneath the skin of the temples. The name comes from the abnormally large cells that develop in the blood vessel walls (see left).

The first symptom is usually a headache, sometimes severe, on one or both sides of the head. Affected arteries may be swollen and the scalp tender. The condition can occur at the same time as polymyalgia rheumatica.

Giant cell arteritis needs rapid treatment as complications can set in, the most serious of which is permanent blindness in one or both eyes. Drugs to reduce the inflammation are usually effective, although some people need to take steroids for several years to control the condition.

Osteoporosis

This condition is very different from arthritis because the bones lose their density and become weak and brittle. However, it can be an added complication for people who already have arthritis.

Bones normally maintain their structure by creating cells called osteoblasts, then breaking them down. The process continues throughout life. As people age, their bone cells are broken down faster than they are replaced and their skeleton becomes lighter and more porous.

Osteoporosis affects everyone to some extent as they age and the production of sex hormones, essential for bone maintenance, starts to decline. Women are particularly susceptible once they have reached the menopause because their levels of oestrogen fall rapidly as their ovaries cease production (see p.192).

Just as exercise can help to build up the strength of your bones, so people who remain bedridden or inactive for long periods because of illness can lose bone mass very quickly. Some drug treatments, particularly steroids, that are used for a long time can also speed up the loss of bone density.

Osteoporosis does not in itself cause pain, but it does increase the likelihood of fractures. In fact, the first sign of weakened bones is usually a fracture, often following a comparatively minor fall. In older people, common sites of fracture are the wrist or hip.

If osteoporosis affects the spine, the back may become rounded with a noticeable loss of height. When the vertebrae become seriously weakened, a fracture of one or more of them may occur spontaneously, which causes severe back pain.

Once you have lost bone mass you can no longer replace it. Your doctor may recommend drugs to slow the further progress of osteoporosis and to minimize the risk of fractures. In the meantime, there are a variety of preventive measures that you can take to protect yourself against further bone loss (see p.194).

When treatment for osteoporosis is needed your doctor normally prescribes bisphosphonates, which include alendronic acid and residronate sodium. These may sometimes cause stomach problems in the elderly. Calcitonin is less frequently used.

As people age, their bone cells are broken down faster than they are replaced and their skeleton becomes lighter and more porous.

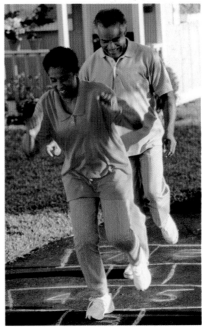

HIGH-IMPACT EXERCISE
Building up the strength of your bones with high-impact exercise can help to prevent osteoporosis – and it can also be enjoyable.

Symptoms and diagnosis

For most people with arthritis, pain is the most immediate predominant symptom. Other symptoms, such as stiffness and inflammation, are due either to the disease itself or to its consequences. When a rheumatologist looks at all your symptoms together, a particular pattern emerges that will help to narrow down and identify the type of arthritis that is affecting you. Such diagnoses are often determined and confirmed by a range of techniques – from X-rays to blood tests – at the rheumatologist's disposal.

The impact of arthritis is to make people less able to live normally and more likely to be disabled.

Recognizing arthritis

Symptoms vary enormously from person to person, depending on both the type of arthritis and its extent and severity. Symptoms are also greatly influenced by personal factors unique to the individual. The key symptoms for recognizing arthritis are pain, inflammation, stiffness, loss of function, joint damage, and fatigue.

Pain
The dominant symptom in all types of arthritis, and indeed in every type of musculoskeletal disease, is pain. Inflamed joints are painful at rest and when they are moved. People with arthritis usually seek medical advice because they want treatment to relieve the pain in their joints.

The subjective sensation of pain in arthritis is very personal. It affects different people in different ways. The exact description of the nature of the pain does not help in the diagnosis of the condition.

Unlike many forms of pain, the pain of arthritis can be chronic, which means that it is present most of the time and lasts for long periods. People with long-term pain experience all sorts of other effects, such as depression.

In arthritis, pain is normally associated with joint tenderness: when a joint is pressed it hurts. The more active the arthritis, the more joints are tender. The number of tender joints provides a good indication of the severity of the arthritis.

Inflammation and swelling

A joint that is inflamed becomes swollen. If the lining of the joint swells, the inflamed joint has synovitis. If the synovial fluid increases in volume the inflamed joint has an effusion.

Inflammation in a joint is the same as inflammation elsewhere in the body. It is an active process in which inflammatory cells (mainly white cells) and more blood enter into the joint. At the same time, many inflammatory molecules, such as small proteins (peptides), are released into the soft tissues around the joint.

The increased blood flow makes the joint swell and feel warm. The inflammatory materials cause fluid to collect in and around the joint, which adds to the swelling.

Stiffness

Inflamed joints can feel stiff first thing in the morning. How long this stiffness lasts is important – an hour or more is highly suggestive of arthritis. Defining morning stiffness is hard, although people with arthritis describe it as an ache combined with difficulty moving.

Stiffness following exercise is usually a feature of osteoarthritis; it is a sign that the joints are starting to fail. People with arthritis may also feel stiff when they rest, such as sitting down after a walk or relaxing in the evening. The joints are sometimes said to "gel", a term reminiscent of how gelatine sets – in other words, a gradual process of firming up.

Loss of function

When joints are painful, swollen, and stiff they start to lose their function, which means they do

IDENTIFYING SYMPTOMS

Pain, inflammation, swelling, and stiffness are the four symptoms that doctors look for when trying to identify arthritis. Sometimes, these symptoms are accompanied by other features, such as loss of function and a sensation of unbearable tiredness, or general symptoms that affect the body as a whole.

SYMPTOMS	WHAT THEY MEAN
Pain	Pain in a joint or joints may be mild, moderate, or severe, and is usually chronic. Joint pain is a symptom of all types of arthritis.
Inflammation	Inflammation is a symptom of the various types of inflammatory arthritis, as well as many instances of osteoarthritis.
Swelling	Either the lining of the joint swells or fluid flows into the joint. Usually indicates inflammatory arthritis.
Stiffness	Morning stiffness that lasts for over an hour usually indicates a form of arthritis. Stiffness that follows exercise usually suggests osteoarthritis.

A complex and subtle issue is the way arthritis can change people's appearance and the way they look at themselves.

Symptoms of pain, tenderness, and swelling provide clues about the nature and extent of arthritis. A doctor will check certain joints, such as the elbow, to see if any of the symptoms are present.

not work well or move properly. As a result, everyday tasks become hard to complete. Arthritis of the hands may cause difficulty with cooking and eating, while arthritis of the knees and feet causes difficulty with walking.

The ways in which arthritis can affect an individual are relative and depend on many circumstances. For example, a previously fit person may be less disabled than an unfit person.

Losing the function of a joint is also a subjective experience; what some people find an inconvenience may to others represent a personal disaster. This does not merely mean that some people cope well with the problems that come with arthritis whilst others do not. It is more complicated than that. For example, a professional musician who plays the violin or piano would find arthritis of the hands far more of a problem than someone who spends their time talking to others without the need for physical performance.

Changes in self-perception

A complex and subtle issue is the way arthritis can change people's appearance and the way they look at themselves. How we look is of fundamental importance to us all. In the long term, arthritis affects both self-image and actual appearance, with consequent changes in self-perception. While these are difficult to quantify, they change a person's quality of life rather than cause a distinct disability, and are important end results of arthritis.

Joint damage

Inflammation that persists can cause damage to an arthritic joint. Eventually, the damage becomes irreversible and the joints look distinctly different. The final common pathway of the damage is one of osteoarthritis and joint failure, but the early stages differ between the types of arthritis and the joints affected.

Damage to cartilage and bone is also accompanied by damage to tendons and soft tissues around joints. This may not be obvious at first, but later it can cause very typical abnormalities. For example, in rheumatoid arthritis tendon damage causes a number of specific changes in the fingers, such as the "swan-neck" deformity.

Fatigue

A marked feature of arthritis is a sensation of unbearable tiredness. It is closely related to pain and to the reduction of mood or even depression, which is commonplace in arthritis. The fatigue is due to poor sleep, weakened muscles, and a disease process that affects the whole body and mind.

General symptoms

Extensive joint inflammation –
for example, in severe rheumatoid
arthritis – may be accompanied by
a low-grade fever, loss of weight,
and a feeling of being generally
unwell. This is because the illness
affects the whole body.

Rashes are a feature in a few
types of arthritis, such as psoriatic
arthritis and lupus. However, in
most people they are a relatively
common side-effect of treatment.

Diagnosing arthritis

After first assessing your personal
circumstances and health status,
your doctor can recommend
various blood tests and imaging
techniques, such as magnetic
resonance imaging (MRI) scans
(see right), to help confirm – or
dispense with – a diagnosis of a
particular type of arthritis.

History and examination

Your doctor will assess you by
listening to your story (the history)
and looking at what is wrong
(the examination) with you.

Your history has a number of
features: the history of the arthritis
itself; general problems; current
and previous treatments; details
of past diseases; the occurrence
of arthritis in your relatives; and
your work and social situation.
The examination will focus on
your joints in particular.

MRI SCANNING

Examination of a joint, such
as the knee, with a magnetic
resonance imaging (MRI)
scan can reveal the extent of
osteoarthritis. A MRI scan literally
takes an image of a slice of your
body and reveals soft tissues that
are not normally visible on X-rays.
The MRI scan of a knee joint
(below) belongs to a man who
developed osteoarthritis at the
unusually early age of 33. The
scan shows the lower end of the
thigh bone (femur) and the upper
end of the shin bone (tibia). Due
to osteoarthritis the bone tissue
at the end of the thigh bone has
become eroded and jagged.
Cracks that have opened up at
the ends of both the bones will
weaken the joint.

MRI SCANNER
A magnetic resonance imaging (MRI)
scanner houses a large magnet that
can make images of slices of your
body. You need to lie very still on
a narrow table inside a tunnel. If
you are concerned about feeling
claustrophobic, make sure your
doctor knows so that you can be
given a sedative.

Knee cap
(patella)

Synovium

Shin bone
(tibia)

MRI SCAN OF A KNEE
The hard and soft features
of the knee are distinctly
revealed by an MRI scan.

Crack at the end of the
thigh bone reveals the
presence of osteoarthritis.

Muscle

ARTHROSCOPY AND BIOPSY

Fibre-optic arthroscopes, which are small and flexible, can look inside large joints, such as the knee, and small joints, such as the wrist. For example, arthroscopy of the knee can distinguish between problems that are due to meniscus damage (torn knee cartilage) and problems resulting from arthritis. Arthroscopes can also be used to obtain a biopsy of the synovial fluid of any joint as a way of checking for infections, crystals, and cells.

ARTHROSCOPY
With a fibre-optic arthroscope, a surgeon can examine a joint very thoroughly and precisely identify a problem.

To the uninitiated it might seem that clinicians ask a whole series of questions, complete a full examination, and then reach a conclusion. In practice, the situation is quite different. If an expert clinician does not have a fairly good idea of the likely diagnosis within a minute or two of talking to you, it will probably be difficult to reach a diagnosis at a later stage.

Most of your history is taken down as a way of ensuring that there is sufficient information to confirm first suspicions about the diagnosis and gaining information about you to recommend the most appropriate treatment.

The examination rarely helps the diagnosis, but instead aids the evaluation of disease severity and pinpoints problems with specific joints. It is also more of an art than a science; there is often disagreement between experts on what may seem the simplest of possible questions, such as whether a joint is swollen or not.

X-rays

Plain radiographs (X-rays) are the classic method of imaging joints. They demonstrate joint damage and can provide a readily available assessment of its severity and progression. They can show loss of bone in arthritis, which in essence means the presence of erosions next to the margins of joints – a characteristic of rheumatoid arthritis.

X-rays also show where there are increases in bone, in particular the presence of osteophytes (bony spurs) in osteoarthritis and loss of cartilage. X-rays can help a doctor decide whether or not joint replacement surgery is needed.

Other imaging techniques

There are a number of other ways of scanning the joints, such as computerized tomography (CT), magnetic resonance imaging (MRI), ultrasound, isotope bone scans, and dual energy X-ray absorptiometry (DEXA). Some, particularly MRI and ultrasound, can show inflammation and soft-tissue swelling. Others, especially DEXA, show the presence of osteoporosis (see p.35).

Many techniques provide improved imaging of bones and joints compared to X-rays. More technically demanding and more expensive than routine radiology, they are, at present, used only in a minority of cases. This could rise rapidly and, in the next 10 years, they will probably replace X-rays for most imaging of joints.

Blood tests

Analysis of the blood can help to confirm a diagnosis or indicate disease severity. The tests are never diagnostic in their own right. They are often used to assess the safety and effectiveness of treatment, too.

■ **ASSESSING THE BODY'S RESPONSE**
Blood tests can assess the normal

way in which the body responds to a damaging situation, such as an infection. In some forms of arthritis, especially rheumatoid arthritis, the response is switched on when it should not be. This response can be detected when the erythrocyte sedimentation rate (ESR) increases (see right).

■ **TESTING FOR MARKERS** Blood tests can look for specific chemicals that are markers of arthritis. The main test of this type measures uric acid levels in the blood serum. These are usually, but not necessarily, raised in people with gout. However, it is also true that in most individuals with a high uric acid level there is no evidence of gout. In addition, in an acute attack of gout, serum uric acid levels may be normal.

■ **TESTING FOR AUTO-ANTIBODIES** Blood tests can identify specific auto-antibodies, such as rheumatoid

factor (see below). Auto-antibodies are antibodies that react with specific proteins in your own body. They are thought to be the by-products of a disturbed immune system, which is a common feature in rheumatoid arthritis and some connective tissue diseases.

However, there is a paradox. The presence of auto-antibodies does not mean that one or other of these diseases is present; indeed, most people with an auto-antibody do not have arthritis. In addition, their absence does not rule out any disease. Nevertheless, most people with an inflammatory arthritis (such as rheumatoid arthritis) or a connective tissue disease, such as lupus, will have an auto-antibody detectable in their blood. The higher the level of auto-antibodies, the greater the chance of having severe disease.

■ **ANTINUCLEAR ANTIBODIES**
Antinuclear antibodies react with components of the normal cell nucleus. They are characteristic of lupus, but also occur in most other connective tissue diseases, rheumatoid arthritis, and other generalized chronic inflammatory conditions. They are a family of different auto-antibodies rather than a single and distinct auto-antibody, and as a result they are very non-specific. Nevertheless, it is usual for people with lupus to have some detectable antinuclear antibodies in their blood.

Q&A

What is rheumatoid factor?

Rheumatoid factor is the best-known auto-antibody and can be detected by blood tests. It reacts with proteins that are released by the immune system. It is detected in about two-thirds of people with rheumatoid arthritis, although its presence in the blood does not necessarily confirm rheumatoid arthritis because it can be associated with other diseases, too. The test for rheumatoid factor is only useful as a diagnostic test when considered with other tests.

ERYTHROCYTE SEDIMENTATION

Red cells (erythrocytes) in a blood sample settle when left to stand. The erythrocyte sedimentation (ESR) test measures how fast they do this. The quicker they settle, the higher the ESR and the more inflammation there is. It is measured in millimetres per hour. Normally, it is less than 20, but is 50–100 in active rheumatoid arthritis. At the same time, there is a small fall in numbers of red cells and changes in specific blood proteins. The most frequently measured protein is the C-reactive protein. This is normally less than 5mg/litre in the blood and in active arthritis can be 50–100mg/litre.

SEDIMENTATION TEST

Looking after your arthritis

There is no need to feel helpless about a diagnosis of arthritis. Today, there are more treatment options available to you than ever before, from drugs and surgery to self-help measures and counselling. But no longer do you have to be a mere recipient of treatment. Increasingly, your input in helping to manage your own arthritis will be welcomed and encouraged by doctors and by many of the other health professionals who may be involved in both diagnosis and treatment.

Building up a working partnership with your doctor will increase your confidence and help you to feel in control of your arthritis.

Working with your healthcare professionals

If you have arthritis, you are likely to need regular health care on a long-term basis. Establishing a good relationship with your doctor and other practitioners, such as physiotherapists and nurses, can go a long way towards reducing the stress and anxiety of coping with treatment and consultations.

Most importantly, mutual trust and understanding between you and your health professionals means that you have the best chance of getting the treatment that is exactly right for you.

Two-way communication

Communication is the key to successful health care. As a patient, you can expect to receive the information you need from your doctor. It is equally important that he or she, in return, receives information from you.

Doctors can learn a great deal about your condition from tests and physical examinations, but there are things they will not necessarily find out unless you tell them. Your personal knowledge of how arthritis – and its treatment – affects you is of value to your doctor. Don't hesitate to share your concerns and feel confident about speaking openly of your needs, symptoms, and feelings. Building up a working partnership with your doctor will increase your confidence and help you to feel in control of your arthritis.

Making the most of your doctor's appointment

Visiting the doctor's surgery or attending a hospital appointment can be daunting, especially if you are newly diagnosed with arthritis. It may help communications to go more smoothly if you take a friend or relative. Another person not only provides moral support if you are nervous, but he or she can also be on hand to assist if you are hard of hearing or do not speak English as your first language.

Doctors work under enormous pressure and most of them have less than 10 minutes in which to see individual patients, so make the best use of their time – and yours – by being well prepared for your appointment. Before you go, make a list of the important questions you want to ask or points you wish to discuss. Keep this list as concise as possible by focusing on the essentials.

Medical terminology can be confusing, so if you do not understand what your doctor tells you, don't hesitate to ask him or her to repeat it or to explain things more simply. If you want more information, say so. Take a notepad with you to write down anything that you need to remember – it is easy to forget what has been said once you leave the surgery or consulting room. If you run out of time to discuss everything you want, ask for another appointment.

PRACTICAL TIPS

WHAT YOU CAN DO

● Keep a diary to monitor your progress and the effects of any treatment. It will provide a handy record to discuss with your health professionals.

● If you are not satisfied with your health care, tell your doctor – this will not cause offence.

● Don't be afraid to suggest alternative treatments to your doctor, but be guided by his or her advice.

● When talking to your health professionals, be honest about how arthritis affects your personal life and emotional well-being.

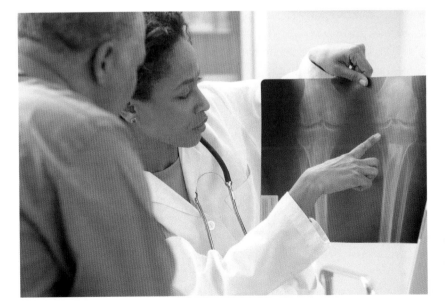

DISCUSSING YOUR ARTHRITIS
An appointment with your doctor is the best opportunity you have to discuss your arthritis and to communicate your thoughts and feelings about the condition.

PRACTICAL TIPS

SELF-HELP STRATEGIES

You may find that drugs or surgery alone are not able to keep your arthritis in check. Regardless of whether you need extra medical help, the following self-help strategies will make a difference and almost certainly improve your quality of life overall. They may even bring some relief from symptoms such as pain and inflammation.

● Make changes to your lifestyle.

● Think positively about your arthritis.

● Take exercise (see p.64) or practise exercise sequences (see p.158).

● Learn to cope with your stress (see p.152).

● Eat well (see p.50).

● Practise relaxation and meditation (see p.156).

● A complementary therapy (see pp.108–131) may also help you to take control of your arthritis.

Getting the best from your treatment

Try to take an active role in your arthritis management plan by learning about different treatment options and what you can expect from them. Being informed means being more involved in decisions regarding your health care.

Management of arthritis differs from person to person, according to the severity of the condition and factors such as how individuals tolerate certain drugs. What suits one may not work so well with another – so make sure that your health professionals are aware of your personal needs and concerns. The more a doctor knows about you and your lifestyle, the more precisely he or she can tailor treatment to your particular requirements.

Keep your doctor up to date with aspects of your treatment that affect your quality of life. For example, your medication may be causing unacceptable side-effects or your exercise programme may prove too strenuous. A prompt word means that you and your doctor can work together to prevent small problems turning into bigger ones. At the same time, you should also report the good news of any improvements.

Be a considerate patient

Your relationship with healthcare professionals will benefit if your expectations are reasonable.

Always arrive on time for an appointment; if you have to cancel, tell the surgery or hospital as soon as you can. Don't demand appointments at short notice or ask your doctor to make home visits unless there is urgent need. If you are on repeat prescriptions, make sure that you request a repeat before you run out of tablets. Last-minute panics are unwelcome interruptions to busy doctors and their staff.

Your treatment options

The kind of treatment you and your doctor decide you need will depend on a range of factors, including the type and severity of your arthritis, potential side-effects, and, of course, your own feelings and lifestyle concerns.

Drug treatment

A wide variety of drugs may be prescribed by doctors or bought over the counter at pharmacies. These include analgesics, non-specific anti-inflammatory drugs (NSAIDs), steroids, disease-modifying anti-rheumatic drugs (DMARDs), and biologic agents (see pp.76–87).

Over-the-counter medicines

Many analgesics (see p.77) and NSAIDs (see p.78) are available over the counter, but in lower doses than those your doctor

would prescribe. All other drugs
for arthritis are available only on
prescription. Always read the
information carefully and make
sure you take the correct dosage.
Over-the-counter medicines can be
dangerous if not taken properly.

Generic vs. brand drugs

All medicines have an approved,
or generic, name. Paracetamol and
ibuprofen are examples of generic
names. These are the ones that
doctors will generally use. Generic
drugs are also much cheaper than
brand names.

Brands sometimes offer extra
ingredients, although often they
will be identical in composition
to the cheaper generic versions.
There are strict laws in place to
ensure that both generic and
brand-name drugs are equally
effective and safe to use.

Q&A

**Is it safe to buy drugs through
the internet?**

At least 600,000 people in the UK
have bought medicines over the
internet, according to one survey.
However, organizations such as
the British Medical Association have
warned against it. Although there are
genuine online pharmacies, many
have no regulations or controls so
the drugs they offer may not be safe
or of good quality, and vital patient
information may be missing. Only buy
medicines from regular pharmacies
and on the advice of your doctor.

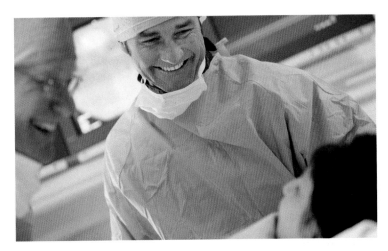

Surgery

When drugs cannot control your
arthritis because of the extensive
damage to the joints involved,
your rheumatologist may suggest
that you undergo surgery (see
pp.88–107). It may take time
to arrange an operation so be
prepared to join a waiting list.

Joint replacement, particularly
of the hips, is common, although
surgeons can also replace joints
in the shoulders, knees, ankles,
elbows, wrists, and fingers. They
can also remove the lining in a
joint, remove bone, and fuse joints
to make them more stable.

MEETING YOUR SURGEON
Before you have surgery to treat
your arthritis you can talk to the
surgeon who will be conducting
the operation.

Professional care

Many different health professionals
may be involved in the diagnosis
and treatment of your arthritis.
Some you may see once only,
others more than once or on an
on-going basis, depending on the
type and severity of your arthritis.

General practitioners

Your GP is your partner in caring for your arthritis and will be your main point of contact for any long-term care. Your GP can examine joints and look for signs of swelling or reduced mobility. He or she can refer you to a nearby hospital for tests or to a specialist.

Rheumatologists

Rheumatologists are hospital-based doctors who have undergone 4 or 5 years specialist training in arthritis and other diseases that affect the joints. You can consult them on the NHS or privately. A rheumatologist can interpret your tests and may suggest more. He or she will discuss treatment and can prescribe drugs or refer you for surgery if that is required.

Children suspected of having arthritis (see p.182), may need to be referred to a paediatric rheumatologist. You and your child may have to travel to see one. Alternatively, a regular rheumatologist may be able to help.

Orthopaedic specialists

Your GP may refer you to an orthopaedic doctor or surgeon who specializes in muscle and bone disorders. They practise in the orthopaedic department of a hospital or in conjunction with the rheumatology department. Orthopaedic surgeons perform joint replacement surgery; some may specialize in particular joints, such as the feet and ankles.

Physiotherapists

A physiotherapist is a specialist in physical treatments that help to restore movement and function in the body. He or she may use a range of different methods, from massage and manipulation to the use of heat and hydrotherapy. At the first session they ask you about your condition and examine you. They may suggest an appropriate course of treatment, which may require further sessions.

Occupational therapists

If your arthritis causes practical problems at home or at work the best person to turn to for help is an occcupational therapist. They are usually based in a hospital or social services department. Ask your GP to refer you or approach the social services department directly. (See also p.144.)

Nurses and nurse practitioners

Nurses at your health centre or at hospital organize blood tests and provide advice on medication, among their many other roles. Nurse practitioners are highly experienced nurses who have

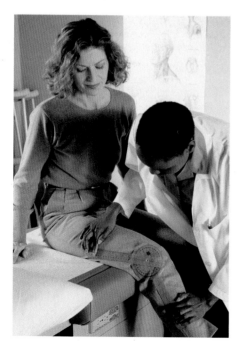

PHYSIOTHERAPY
Physiotherapists may employ various techniques and physical treatments to help people with arthritis restore normal movement to their joints.

extra training that allows them to take on certain roles traditionally carried out only by doctors.

Dietitians and nutritionists

If you need to lose weight, your GP may refer you to a dietitian for advice on what foods are best for you to eat. Dietitians must follow an established training programme and be registered to practise. Nutritionists have a very similar role, but while they may also have undergone proper training they do not need it to set themselves up in business.

Counselling

All doctors agree that pain is a complex and little-understood process and many people believe there is a strong link between the mind and body. By talking things through with a professional counsellor, you may make a very real difference to the level of pain and discomfort you experience.

You can access counselling services on the NHS via your GP. If you consult a counsellor privately, make sure he or she is registered with a recognized body such as the British Association of Counselling and Psychotherapy.

Support groups

These are a good way of keeping up to date on new treatments for arthritis, learning tips on coping with your pain and condition, and getting in touch with others who

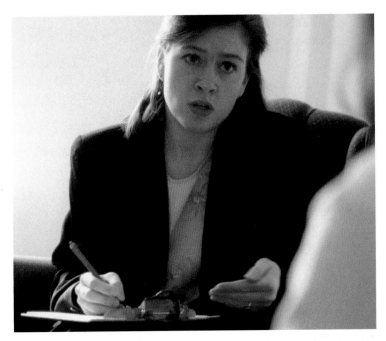

share your experiences or problems. You may have to pay a subscription fee. Most support groups provide helplines or free internet information. Some examples include the British Pain Foundation, the Pain Association Scotland, and Pain Concern (see Useful addresses, p.217).

Pain clinics

Specialist NHS clinics in certain UK hospitals help people deal with their long-term pain. They employ a range of professionals, from nurses and doctors to complementary practitioners, such as acupuncturists, and practise various methods, such as drug injections, hydrotherapy, and pain management programmes. Your GP will be able to locate the nearest pain clinic to you.

COUNSELLING
Healthcare professionals will provide you with all kinds of treatment, advice, and guidance that will help you to look after and manage your arthritis.

Food, drink, and physical activity

Eating a balanced diet and taking regular exercise is good advice for everyone, but it is especially important if you have arthritis. These two crucial aspects of everyday life not only make you feel better but they also help you to manage your weight.

While there is no evidence that specific foods can cure or cause arthritis, medical research suggests that some nutrients, such as omega-3 fatty acids, may be able to help relieve the symptoms. However, the best advice is to follow a diet that is rich in oily fish, fruit, vegetables, and low-fat dairy products, rather than relying on supplements or superfoods.

Regular physical activity and exercise can bring you many benefits. But you don't need to overdo it – just stay within your comfort zone. Your joints will become more mobile and flexible, while the adjacent muscles and other soft tissues remain healthy. Perhaps the best benefit comes from keeping stiffness at bay and bringing some welcome relief from pain.

Eating to ease your arthritis

It is a popular belief that what you eat can relieve the inflammation and pain of arthritis. Some people are also convinced that certain foods can trigger their arthritis attacks. However, in most cases there is no firm medical evidence to confirm this. Your doctor may discourage you from emphasizing the links between food and arthritis, but there are good reasons for paying attention to your diet. As our understanding of arthritis progresses, it is becoming clear that what you eat may have potential benefits.

If you are getting the right nutrients you will maximize your chances of fighting disease.

Food and arthritis

People with arthritis need to eat the type of well-balanced diet that would be a healthy choice for anyone, regardless of his or her age or fitness. As a general guide, meals should include fish, both white and oily types, low-fat dairy products, lots of fresh fruits and vegetables, and only occasional greasy deep-fried foods and sugary treats. Meat-eaters can also have poultry and occasional red meat.

Many unsubstantiated claims have been made for the benefits of eliminating specific foods, or food groups, or focusing on so-called "superfoods" to reduce pain and inflammation, but you should regard these with extreme caution. Dietitians and doctors generally do not recommend such diets, as they could possibly be detrimental to your general health. If you do want to explore the possibilities of special diets consult a registered dietitian first.

What makes up a healthy diet?

Healthy eating means choosing a variety of foods that will supply your body with the energy (calories) it needs to keep all its systems functioning normally. If you are getting the right nutrients you will maximize your chances of fighting disease.

The five essential components of food are: carbohydrates, protein, fats, vitamins, and minerals. You need some of these components in larger quantities than others; the key to a healthy diet is getting the right balance.

Carbohydrates

Carbohydrates are our main source of energy. They are found mainly in starchy foods – such as bread, cereals, rice, pasta, and potatoes – and in sugar. Starchy foods also contain fibre and some nutrients essential to good health, including calcium, iron, and B vitamins. Sugar provides only calories and is of little nutritional value.

Starchy foods should make up about a third of what you eat. Wholegrain or wholemeal varieties of cereals, bread, rice, and pasta are the best options because they contain more fibre than the white varieties. It is fibre that keeps you feeling fuller for longer – it also helps to keep your bowels functioning effectively.

Try to include starchy foods in each main meal. For example, start the day with a wholegrain cereal or freshly prepared porridge. (Some packet varieties of porridge may be full of sugar. If you need a sweetener, add some dried fruit or a banana instead.)

At lunch you could have a sandwich made with wholemeal or wholegrain bread, pitta or chapatti. For your evening meal you could include bread, potatoes (in their skins), pasta, or rice.

MYTH OR TRUTH?

MYTH

Food sensitivities play a major role in provoking the symptoms of arthritis.

TRUTH

Most inflammation is not caused by sensitivity to one particular food or another, although some people do find that certain foods worsen their symptoms. It is better to follow a diet containing foods that are good for your health and may help to lessen inflammation, rather than to focus on potential dietary culprits. Eliminating food groups can deprive your body of important nutrients.

PASTA, PULSES, AND GRAINS
The wide variety of pasta, pulses, and grains provides plenty of choices for ensuring your diet contains enough fibre and protein.

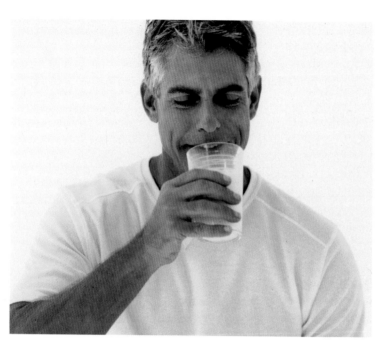

MILK
Dairy products, such as milk, cheese, butter, and yoghurt, are good sources of protein.

teaspoons of sugar in tea and coffee or on cereals, cut down or do without, particularly if you are trying to lose weight (see p.62).

Protein

You need protein to keep every tissue in your body, including bones, muscles, internal organs, and skin, in good working order. Some proteins are produced naturally in body cells; however, most of the protein we need to stay healthy comes from the diet and is found in a wide variety of foods, including fish, poultry, meat, eggs, and dairy products such as cheese, milk, and yoghurt.

Beans (such as red kidney beans and chick peas), pulses (such as lentils and barley), and meat substitutes (such as tofu) are also good sources of protein.

All these foods contain vitamins and minerals essential to good health – for example, iron in red meat and some beans and pulses,

Beans and pulses are good sources of fibre, too. You could also try adding chick peas or green lentils to salads or making a chilli con carne with extra kidney beans and cut down on the red meat.

If you are not used to eating much fibre, introduce it gradually to your diet by using both white and high-fibre foods. For example, start with a small wholemeal or wholegrain loaf and just use it for toast at breakfast (you can keep the loaf in the freezer). Try adding a high-fibre cereal, such as muesli or bran flakes, to your usual one.

Cakes and pastries usually contain a lot of white flour and sugar and fat, so are full of calories that you probably don't need. Eat them only occasionally as a lot of sugar is not good for your health. If you use more than a couple of

Q&A

Should I avoid cow's milk because it contains too much protein and drink soya milk instead?

There is no need to avoid cow's milk – if you do you will reduce your intake of calcium, which is vital for strong, healthy bones. Soya milk does not have calcium unless the manufacturer has added it. If you continue to use soya milk make sure to buy one that is fortified with calcium.

calcium in dairy products. Most people need only two portions of protein-rich food a day, as well as the milk in cereal, tea, and coffee. A 100g portion of roast chicken has 25g protein, 120g of salmon fillet has 15g of protein, 2 eggs have 12g of protein, 50g tofu has 11g of protein, and 230g of cooked pasta has 9g of protein.

A flare-up of arthritis, especially rheumatoid arthritis, can cause muscle weakness and weight loss, but it can also make you feel generally unwell and lose your appetite. So you might need to eat smaller protein-rich meals more frequently to get the amount of protein you need.

Fats and oils

All fats and oils are high in energy and they are essential to the body's absorption of certain vitamins. They come in different forms and some are more beneficial to your health than others, so it is important to know what kind of fat you are eating.

The type known as saturated fat is found in red meat and many processed foods – for example, meat pies, sausages, hard cheese, butter, cakes, pastry, cream, coconut oil, and palm oil. This saturated fat is not regarded as a "healthy" fat because eating large amounts can increase the level of cholesterol in your blood and contribute to having a higher risk of developing heart disease.

Unsaturated fats in vegetable oils, some margarines, and oily fish are generally better for you and your heart. Today, there is so much choice it is not difficult or expensive to eat fats that may be more beneficial, particularly for people with arthritis.

Try to cut down on foods that are high in saturated fats and eat more that are rich in unsaturated fats. These include rapeseed, sunflower, and olive oils, oily fish, avocados, and some nuts (such as almonds and pecan). (See p.56 for information on omega-3 fatty acids, which may help ease arthritis.)

AVOCADO
Eating an avocado in a salad will help you boost your intake of unsaturated fats and cut down on saturated fats.

SPINACH
If you don't like to eat dairy products, spinach and other dark-green, leafy vegetables are also good sources of calcium.

Vitamins and minerals

Most of the fresh foods we eat contain naturally occurring vitamins and minerals, which all work in different ways and do highly specialized jobs to keep the body functioning normally. We need some vitamins and minerals in only tiny amounts, while we need to take in more of others.

Most people obtain sufficient vitamins and minerals from a varied diet, but if you avoid certain foods, or groups of foods, you could miss out on a specific vitamin or mineral. For example, if you don't eat dairy products or take supplements you may not get sufficient calcium, a mineral vital for strong, healthy bones.

Fluids

Water is essential to life – 60 to 70 per cent of your body is made up of water – so don't forget to take in plenty of fluids. You should try to drink 6 to 8 glasses (about 1.5 litres) of fluid a day.

If you have difficulty drinking plain water there are healthy alternatives, such as flavoured water and fruit juice. You should drink tea and coffee only in moderate amounts. Some people believe that water or other fluid helps arthritis by lubricating the joints. This is not true, but too little fluid can lead to dehydration, which will make you feel generally unwell and could lead to or exacerbate attacks of gout.

WATER
Drinking water helps to replace the water that a body loses via breathing, urine, and perspiration.

Salt

While salt is vital for maintaining the balance of water in the body, eating too much of it can be harmful – it can raise your blood pressure, for example. If you already have high blood pressure, eating excessive amounts of salt could put you at increased risk of further complications, such as heart disease or stroke.

Approximately 75 per cent of the salt that we eat comes from processed food, such as ready-prepared meals, soups, sauces, and even some breakfast cereals. You could easily be eating too much salt already without realizing it. (See Fat and Salt, right, for information on assessing the amount of salt in a food product.)

Adults and children over the age of 11 should have no more than 6g (about a teaspoon) of salt a day. The following tips should help if you want to cut down on your intake of salt:

• Try to eat as much fresh food as you possibly can.

• Add no more than a pinch of salt to your cooking.

• Taste your food before adding more salt at the table – you probably don't need it.

Alcohol

There is nothing wrong with having the occasional alcoholic drink. But alcohol is high in calories and regular drinking can contribute to weight gain.

FAT AND SALT

The information on food labels does not always make it clear whether a product contains high or low levels of fat and salt. The explanations given below will help you to work out whether the food you are buying is a healthy option.

WHAT IS IT?	WHAT DOES IT MEAN?
Fat Generally, the label will say how many grams (g) of fat there are in 100g of the food. Some foods also give a separate figure for saturated fat, or "saturates".	• This is A LOT of fat: 20g fat or more per 100g 5g saturates or more per 100g • This is A LITTLE fat: 3g fat or less per 100g 1g saturates or less per 100g Between 3g and 20g per 100g of a food is a moderate amount of *total fat*. Between 1g and 5g is a moderate amount of *saturates*. Try to choose more foods that only contain a little fat (3g fat or less per 100g) and cut down on foods that contain a lot of fat (20g fat or more per 100g).
Salt Salt is often listed on food labels as sodium. A gram (g) of sodium = 2.5g of salt.	• This is A LOT of salt: 1.25g salt or more per 100g 0.5g sodium or more per 100g • This is A LITTLE salt: 0.25g salt or less per 100g 0.1g sodium or less per 100g Try to choose foods that are low in salt (0.25g salt or less per 100g).

Excessive quantities of alcohol can, in the long term, seriously damage your health and put you at significant risk of liver disease, cardiovascular disorders, and some cancers. Alcohol is also known to provoke or exacerbate painful attacks of gout, so it is probably best to avoid alcoholic drinks if you are frequently affected by this condition.

PRACTICAL TIPS

UNITS OF ALCOHOL

The alcoholic content of a drink is measured by the percentage of alcohol by volume (ABV). The following is a guide to standard measures. If you drink at home these measures are unlikely to be exact.

- 1 unit = half a pint of beer/lager/cider (3–5 per cent ABV) or a single measure of spirits (40 per cent ABV).

- 1.5 units = one alcopop (5 per cent ABV).

- 2 units = a small (175ml) glass of wine (11.5–14.5 per cent ABV – the higher the ABV, the more units of alcohol).

If you do drink alcohol, try to keep to the recommended number of units per week. For men, this should be no more than 3 units a day (21 units per week) and for women, no more than 2 units a day (14 units per week). See Units of alcohol (left), which shows you how many units of alcohol are in some of our favourite tipples.

If you are a wine drinker, keep an eye on the alcohol content percentage – it can make a big difference to the number of units you drink. If you have gout, especially avoid alcoholic drinks that contain sediment, such as real ale, mature red wine, or port.

Finally, make sure you have at least two alcohol-free days a week to give your liver a rest, and – above all – avoid binge drinking.

Nutrients that may help your arthritis

By eating a varied diet that includes plenty of fresh foods, you can be sure that you will get enough of every nutrient that is essential to keep you in good general health. However, people with arthritis may benefit from boosting their intake of certain foods and nutrients. (See also Natural Remedies and Supplements, pp.112–119, for further information on adding supplements to your diet.)

WALNUTS
If you don't like eating fish, walnuts are a good alternative source of omega-3 fatty acids.

Omega-3 fatty acids

Polyunsaturated fatty acids are a group of fats that may benefit people with arthritis. One form of these – known as omega-3 fatty acids – has been found to reduce both pain and inflammation in people with rheumatoid arthritis.

The foods that contain omega-3 fatty acids are mainly oily fish such as mackerel, salmon, trout, sardines, pilchards, herring, whitebait, and eel. (White fish contains very little of the omega-3 fatty acids, although it is a good source of lean protein.)

Other sources of omega-3 are plant oils, such as rapeseed and safflower, as well as linseeds and walnuts. Omega-3 fatty acids have other health benefits, too. They are good for your heart as well as your joints, and fish oil is a rich source of vitamin D, which is vital for healthy bones.

Q&A

Can plant oils help to relieve some of the symptoms of my rheumatoid arthritis?

The role that plant oils, such as olive oil, play in fighting arthritis has aroused a great deal of interest. A study has shown that people who consume more olive oil are less likely to develop rheumatoid arthritis. However, there is no evidence that taking lots of olive oil can ease the symptoms of rheumatoid arthritis to the same extent that fish oils can.

OILY FISH
Salmon and other oily fish, such as herring, trout, mackerel, and sardines, are good sources of omega-3 fatty acids.

There have been food scares in recent years about oily fish having high levels of pollutant chemicals, such as mercury, dioxins, and PCBs. Current advice from the UK Food Standards Agency suggests that adults can safely eat two to four portions of oily fish a week. One portion is about 140g of fish.

However, women planning to become pregnant should limit their intake of oily fish to one portion a week. Don't eat more than one portion a week of shark, swordfish, or marlin because of the high levels of mercury they may contain (pregnant women should avoid them altogether).

Taking supplements is an easy way of increasing your intake of omega-3 fatty acids, but check the labels or ask the pharmacist for advice if you are not sure what to buy. Oils from the body of the fish contain the most omega-3 fatty acids and are likely to be the most effective supplement for people with arthritis, particularly rheumatoid arthritis.

Cod liver oil contains far less omega-3 fatty acids than fish body oils. Cod liver oils usually have high concentrations of vitamins A and D. Both these vitamins are good for you but too much may be harmful. If you take cod liver oil, limit the dose to one capsule a day and avoid taking other supplements that contain high amounts of vitamin A.

MYTH OR TRUTH?

MYTH

Some foods cause a flare-up in rheumatoid arthritis.

TRUTH

Not necessarily. Common culprits are said to be foods from the nightshade family (potato, onion, tomato, and aubergine) and various peppers and pepper-derived spices (paprika or cayenne). However, studies show that while food-related flares can occur, only a small percentage of people are affected, and so such reactions are most likely to be coincidental.

Should I avoid eating oranges and tomatoes because of the risk that the acid will cause the rheumatoid arthritis in my joints to flare up?

Many people with arthritis think that citrus fruits and tomatoes cause their joints to become inflamed. However, there really is no good evidence that avoiding these foods works for everyone with rheumatoid arthritis. What you do miss out on are tasty foods that are valuable sources of vitamin C and folic acid.

Fruit, vegetables, and antioxidants

Nutrients called antioxidants can prevent or slow the deterioration of healthy tissue that results from exposure to the environment. They are essential to your diet and are especially important if you have arthritis (or want to prevent it).

Most brightly coloured fruits and vegetables contain antioxidants. Good sources include oranges, kiwi fruit, sweet corn, blueberries, cranberries, red grapes, prunes, broccoli, spinach, carrots, and tomatoes. Green tea (see p.118) is also rich in antioxidants and some research has shown that it may be particularly good for people with osteoarthritis.

FRUIT AND VEGETABLES
A regular daily intake of fresh fruit and vegetables is essential for health because of the vitamins, minerals, and antioxidants they contain.

Bananas, mushrooms, and tomatoes are good sources of potassium, a mineral that helps muscles to work properly and contributes to maintaining healthy bones and reducing the risk of osteoporosis. Some prescribed drugs for arthritis can lower the level of potassium in the blood, so including potassium-rich foods in your diet can help to prevent this.

Five a day
Try to eat at least five portions of fruit and vegetables a day. As a rough guide, one portion equals:
- An apple, orange, grapefruit, pear, or banana.
- Two plums or kiwi fruit.
- A slice of melon or pineapple.
- Three heaped tablespoons of mixed fruit salad.
- A heaped tablespoon of dried fruit.
- 150ml of pure fruit juice.
- Eight cherry tomatoes.
- Three heaped tablespoons of vegetables, such as beans.
- A bowl of salad as a side serving.

Eating five portions might be easier than you think – just add up what you eat during the day. You could have:
- A glass of juice and a sliced banana with your cereal at breakfast (two portions).
- A side salad at lunch (one portion).
- A pear as an afternoon snack (one portion).
- A serving of vegetables with your evening meal (one portion).

PRACTICAL TIPS

MAKING THE MOST OF FRUIT AND VEGETABLES

- Eat fruit and vegetables that are as fresh as possible.
- Always cover and chill cut-up vegetables. Don't soak them, as vitamins and minerals can be lost.
- Don't overcook fruit and vegetables. Start with boiling water and cover the pan tightly to keep in the steam and speed up the cooking. You could also use a steamer or a microwave.
- Cook fruit and vegetables in a little water and then use the water to make sauce or soup.
- Don't leave cooked fruit or vegetables standing hot for too long because the vitamin levels start to drop within a few minutes.

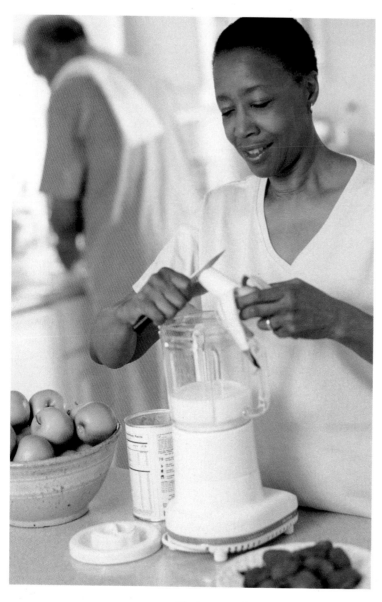

BANANA SMOOTHIE
Fruit smoothies served straight from the blender are brimming with goodness and make an excellent way to start the day

Dairy products and calcium
Dietitians strongly recommend that everyone, especially women, should regularly eat foods that are rich in the mineral calcium – ideally, from childhood through to old age – to keep their bones healthy and prevent osteoporosis (see p.35) later in life.

Good sources of calcium include dairy products (such as milk, yogurt, and cheese), certain dried fruits (such as apricots), green leafy vegetables (such as spinach and cabbage), pulses, sesame seeds, and sardines with their bones. You should try to include some of these foods in your diet on a daily basis.

Malic acid and magnesium
Some unconfirmed evidence suggests that high doses of malic acid and magnesium supplements may bring relief for people with fibromyalgia who have all-over muscle pain. Apples are a source of both nutrients. Magnesium may interact with the medication you are taking so check with your doctor before taking high doses.

Folic acid
Folic acid, which is also known as folate, belongs to the B group of vitamins. This nutrient can help to alleviate the side-effects of some of the medications for rheumatoid arthritis, such as methotrexate and sulphasalazine (see p.84). To counteract these side-effects a high dose of folic acid supplements is usually prescribed once a week.

You can also boost your natural intake of folic acid by eating a whole range of foods. These include green leafy vegetables (such as cabbage, spinach, and Brussels sprouts), beans, whole grains, wholemeal bread, fortified

Q&A

I have been avoiding certain foods for six months now and am not sure it's helping. How can I tell if this elimination diet works, and should I keep to it?

If you're not sure that avoiding the foods has helped, try adding them back into your diet one at a time – say once a week. Keep a diary of what you eat and make a note of any symptoms you feel. This way you may be able to tell if any of the foods are making you feel worse. If yes, then continue to avoid that food but otherwise put them all back into your diet and enjoy eating them.

breakfast cereals, liver, yeast extract, egg yolk, as well as milk and other dairy products.

Vitamin E and selenium

Vitamin E (found in wheatgerm, vegetable oils, nuts, and seeds) and the mineral selenium, found in Brazil nuts (one nut contains your daily intake of selenium), meat, and cereals, may benefit people with rheumatoid arthritis. Current research is not conclusive enough to suggest that taking these supplements is advisable. If you take them, make sure they come from natural sources and don't exceed the recommended dose.

Purine-rich foods and gout

Some foods contain high levels of substances called purines, which, when broken down in the body

during digestion can cause an increase in uric acid. Excess uric acid deposited in joint tissues is the cause of the severe pain felt in gout (see p.23).

Many foods are rich in purines. These include offal (liver, kidneys, heart, haggis, and black pudding), meat extract; hung game (such as venison, extra mature beef, grouse, and duck); some oil-rich fish (such as mackerel, herring, shellfish, and anchovies); yeast (extract and tablets); and hard, extra mature cheese.

Unfortunately, many of these purine-rich foods are also highly nutritious; some, such as the oily fish, are recommended for inflammatory conditions such as rheumatoid arthritis.

If you are prone to repeated attacks of gout, particularly if your symptoms are not controlled by

High doses of malic acid and magnesium supplements may bring relief for people with fibromyalgia who have all-over muscle pain.

EGGS
The yolk of an egg contains a number of vitamins such as folic acid and vitamin B12 that are essential for health.

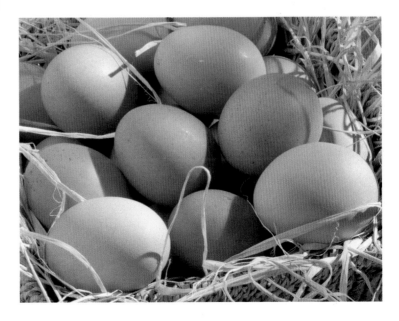

medication, then avoiding these purine-rich foods may help you to keep acute attacks at bay.

Alcohol, especially beer, is also high in purines, so restrict how much you drink – or better still, cut out alcohol altogether.

Weight control

One of the most important things you can do is to keep your weight within a healthy range. Being either too fat or too thin not only affects how well you manage your arthritis but also has implications for other aspects of your health. There is no such thing as the "ideal" weight. The weight that is right for you depends on various factors, such as your height, age, and level of activity.

Always speak to your doctor before embarking on a programme to lose or gain weight, because your medication and any other treatments may need to be adjusted accordingly. If you are a healthy weight now (see BMI, p.199), then try and keep it that way by eating sensibly and staying as active as possible.

Being overweight

If you are overweight you could be helping to making your arthritis worse, as you will be putting extra stress on your joints. Excess fat is also thought be directly linked to the process of inflammation, so

CRUDITÉS
Snack on fruit and raw vegetables such as apples, celery, radishes, and carrot sticks, instead of giving in to the temptation of sweet biscuits and cakes.

people with rheumatoid arthritis should be especially careful to control their weight.

Extreme overweight (obesity) is known to be a major risk factor for developing osteoarthritis, especially of the knees, hips, and hands. Obesity may also mean that joint replacement surgery cannot be considered as an option for treating arthritis. This is because people who are very overweight may be at greater risk when having a general anaesthetic and also because they tend not to do so well after the operation.

Besides affecting the symptoms of your arthritis, carrying excess weight puts an additional strain on your heart and is a major risk factor for serious disorders such as stroke, high blood pressure (hypertension), and diabetes.

Losing excess weight will help you move around more – and keeping active is important in maintaining joint health. Rapid weight loss is not advisable, especially if you have gout; a sudden and severe restriction of your calorie intake can trigger a gouty attack. Fasting is especially dangerous and could leave you weak and undernourished. (For healthy eating suggestions, see Tips for Losing Weight, p.62.)

Being underweight

It isn't healthy to be too thin, because this can lead to problems such as weakened muscles and reduced resistance to infections. Being underweight is common in people with rheumatoid arthritis.

Unwanted weight loss sometimes occurs during a flare-up of the disease, when the metabolism of the body tends to speed up; in addition, feeling generally unwell and the effects of certain drugs can cause loss of appetite.

Elderly people with rheumatoid arthritis are particularly likely to be underweight because they have difficulty using their hands to prepare food and so do not eat enough proper nutrients. (For devices that make preparing and cooking food easier, see p.137.)

Trying to put on weight can sometimes be harder than trying to lose it. If you are not sure what you should be eating, ask your doctor to refer you to a registered dietitian for a diet plan. (For dietary suggestions, see Tips for Gaining Weight, right.)

PRACTICAL TIPS

TIPS FOR GAINING WEIGHT

Eating to gain weight could mean that you risk adding unhealthy levels of fat to your diet, especially if you use full-fat dairy products. Check with your doctor before increasing your intake of fats and oils or following any of the suggestions given below:

● Eat several small meals during the day, rather than attempting (and failing) to eat one or two large ones.

● If you have difficulty facing solid foods, try drinking milkshakes made with fruit or eating soups with added milk or cream.

● Eat nutritious snacks between meals, such as cheese, peanut butter, and dried fruits.

● Eat fish or lean meat every day to boost your protein intake.

● Add butter or cheese sauces to vegetables.

● Don't drink too much fluid immediately before a meal – it can make you feel too full to eat properly.

LEAN MEAT
Stir-fried chicken makes a good meal for people who need to eat lean meat every day in order to gain weight.

Physical activity

Exercise and physical activity are known to be very effective in reducing joint pain and disability. Yet few people with arthritis receive advice about taking exercise and getting involved in physical activity. Your joints and muscles depend on each other to maintain and improve their health and to control your movement. Regular exercise is essential for keeping your joints working efficiently. It may seem like a paradox, but simple physical activities – not rest – can not only keep your joints and muscles working properly but can also contribute to reducing your pain and disability.

Exercise and physical activity help your heart, lungs, and blood vessels become stronger and more efficient, so that you can do more with less effort.

The benefits of physical activity

Movement is good for your joints. Exercise and regular physical activity will ensure that your joints and muscles work efficiently and effectively by making them do what they were designed to do – move, contract, and work.

An increasing amount of evidence indicates that the movement involved in exercise and physical activity has many benefits for people with arthritis. It is able to reduce your pain (see pp.146–151), improve your muscle strength, make you feel less tired, and maintain movement in your joints. It can also help to bring back and maintain your mobility (see pp.158–171).

Exercise and physical activity benefit the rest of your body, too. They strengthen bones, improve breathing and circulation, reduce stress, stimulate digestion, keep body weight down, and encourage better patterns of sleep.

The perils of being inactive

Anyone who stops being active for a prolonged period of time will find that their muscles and bones grow weaker and the cartilage lining their joints becomes thinner.

Is it true that if I don't exercise and remain inactive I will almost certainly have health problems?

Yes. It is difficult to predict exactly what those health problems will be because they vary from one person to another. Exercise and physical activity help your heart, lungs, and blood vessels become stronger and more efficient, so that you can do more with less effort. Other benefits include less cholesterol, better control of diabetes, protection from some forms of cancer, less depression, increased self-confidence, and greater dignity, independence, and self-esteem.

As a result, they feel tired sooner and their joints will stiffen up.

In fact, inactivity is bad for your joints. It causes both stiffness and muscle weakness, which accelerate joint damage, leading to greater pain and disability. "Rest and take things easy" may be sound advice when a joint is very inflamed and painful. However, once the pain and inflammation subside the joint stiffness, pain, muscle weakness, and disability will return and get worse – unless you resume your previous level of activity.

You may intuitively understand that movement is good for your joints – after all, it's what they are designed to do and why you have them. What may concern and confuse you is your experience that activity often causes joint pain and rest eases it. You may interpret your experience as: pain signals joint damage caused by activity and resting prevents joint damage. Understandably, you may assume that reducing physical activity will prolong the life of your joints and make your life more bearable.

Rest, in the short term, may make you feel a bit better. But over time, you will find that everything – especially your mobility and flexibility – gets much worse.

Exercise as part of your treatment

Many people who have arthritis consider the pain in their joints to be an inevitable and incurable consequence of living and aging. Painkilling drugs are, perhaps, the only treatment they have ever really been offered.

Increasingly, people who have arthritis are receiving appropriate advice about the benefits of

DOING EXERCISE
Regular exercise is one of the cornerstones of health as it keeps the body in trim and encourages the mind to be alert.

EXERCISES FOR HEALTHY MUSCLES

These exercises will help you to attain and maintain an adequate range of movement in your joints and improve muscle strength, endurance, and skill:

● To regain the range of movement in a joint, move it to the end of its present range and hold it there so that you feel a slight stretch. Don't stretch it too far.

● To build muscle strength do a few brief but powerful contractions of the muscle against a high resistance, such as an immovable object or a heavy weight.

● To increase muscle endurance do many smaller contractions of the muscle against a low resistance, such as a light weight.

● To improve muscle skill, frequently practise specific activities, just as if you were learning to walk or write. The muscle activity patterns of the movement become ingrained and you can then perform them almost without thinking.

physical activity and exercise in managing their arthritis. Follow-up appointments may help to reassess their condition and to reinforce advice; they may even be invaluable as a means of re-motivation (see p.72).

Relying on other treatments

Many people with arthritis do not realize the benefits of exercise and so rely on other treatments, particularly drugs, to help them manage their arthritis. However, the majority of people either do not like taking drugs, or they experience negative side-effects or have breathing, heart, circulatory, or stomach conditions that prevent them from taking drugs.

Moreover, although drugs can reduce some of the symptoms of arthritis, such as inflammation and pain, they do not alter the underlying condition and nor do they prevent the problems that arthritis can cause, including joint damage, weakness, fatigue, and disability (see p.36).

Surgery can provide an effective last step but it is an option that is usually delayed – and again, many people do not want or cannot have surgery for a variety of health or personal reasons.

All in all, people have to rely on themselves for help. This is not necessarily a bad thing because arthritis is treatable, and there is a great deal you can do to manage your condition and become less

reliant on others. Exercise and physical activity are important parts of the plan.

Exercise and medication

People with inflammatory arthritis, such as rheumatoid arthritis, use medication to help them control their symptoms. Continue to take your prescribed medicine and discuss your exercise needs with your doctor if you wish.

If, however, you have the more common osteoarthritis, ask your doctor if you can reduce the amount of medication you need to control your symptoms. You may be able to take it when you need it to give you most relief, such as before going out, going to bed, or before you exercise. Medication can make your life more comfortable and bearable, and allow you to be physically active.

Separately, drugs and exercise can help; together, they can be very effective. If you start exercising you are still likely to experience times and episodes of pain, but these may not be as often, or as bad, or last as long.

Controlled exercise and even simple physical activity is good for your joints and general health. Whatever you achieve will be hard won by your efforts, but the sense of personal satisfaction and ability to control some of your symptoms will more than compensate.

Range of movement

Each of the joints in your body is designed to move smoothly through a certain range of movement (see p.12). Joints need to be exercised regularly to ensure that their range of movement does not become restricted.

Lack of exercise will probably stop the joint from working effectively and, as a result, it may not respond fully when you need it to. For example, if you cannot bend your knees and hips fully then you will find that walking becomes difficult. If the movement of your shoulder is restricted you will find that combing your hair, washing, and dressing are more difficult. Generally speaking, as you grow older, you lose the range of movement in your joints faster and regain it slower.

Healthy muscles

For your joints to work effectively and efficiently, it is vital that your muscles are in good condition. For a joint to move, one or more of the muscles attached to it need to contract. Yet your muscles do not just bring about large movements, they produce smooth, finely

MUSCLE TONE
Playing a round of golf on a regular basis improves muscle tone and exercises a number of joints in the body.

HOW MUSCLES MOVE A JOINT

Individual skeletal muscles connect two bones together across a joint. A tendon, composed of a tough protein called collagen and wrapped in a synovial sheath, anchors the fibres of a muscle to the fabric of a bone.

Each muscle has the power to contract and exert a pulling force on the bones to which it is attached. Many skeletal muscles, such as the biceps and triceps of the upper arm, are arranged in pairs on either side of a joint. The pairs of muscles work in opposition to make a joint work and move a particular part of the body. For example, the triceps muscle relaxes when the biceps muscle contracts, causing the elbow to bend and moving the lower arm and hand upwards. When the triceps muscle contracts the biceps relaxes, opening the elbow and straightening the arm.

BENDING THE ARM

Humerus

Relaxed triceps muscle

Radius

Ulna

Contracted biceps muscle bends the elbow and pulls up the radius.

Tendon

Relaxed biceps muscle

Humerus

Contracted triceps muscle opens the elbow and straightens the arm.

Tendon

Radius

Ulna

STRAIGHTENING THE ARM

MYTH OR TRUTH?

MYTH

To be effective, exercise must be strenuous.

TRUTH

Doing almost any physical activity regularly is better than doing nothing regularly. On the whole, the more you do the better, but it doesn't have to be hard work.

controlled movements, too. When these two forms of muscle activity are balanced by working together they enable you to be mobile and stable at the same time.

Muscles also provide a warning system by signalling when a joint is moving beyond a safe range of movement. As a result, they can prevent harmful movement and protect against joint injury.

For example, muscles prevent the joints of your legs from jarring as you walk. The activity of the muscles around the weight-bearing joints – your trunk, hips, and knees – enables you to maintain an erect posture as you walk. Yet muscles simultaneously allow you exquisite control of the movement in these joints, enabling you to walk with a smooth gait, without jarring the joints of your legs.

Deconditioned muscles

You need to move muscles to maintain their strength and function. Unfortunately, like the range of movement in your joints, if you do not use your muscle then you lose your muscle. Muscles that are not used regularly become "deconditioned" and unfit – they get smaller, shorter, stiffer, and weaker; they feel heavy and tire quicker during normal activities.

Deconditioned muscles increase the risk of joint sprains, strains, and pains because they are slower to react and so fail to signal when joints are moving out of a safe

range of movement – they are moving too far for comfort. They cannot produce smooth, finely-controlled movements, so you walk with a clumsy, uneven, and jarring gait.

Over time, this can cause pain and damage in your weight-bearing joints, further reducing their function and independence. Therefore, you need to keep your muscles in good condition in order to maintain healthy joints.

Fitting exercise into your life

With so many health benefits, why do so few people with arthritis exercise regularly? Most are never told how beneficial it can be, and the few who are told often receive advice that is unlikely to motivate them to adopt and persevere with a lifestyle change.

We all make excuses for not exercising: "I don't have time" or "It's a burdensome chore" or "It's too much hard work to get the full benefits". Perhaps you think you need expert supervision and access to expensive, sophisticated equipment and facilities.

Acquiring the full health benefits from exercise does undeniably require effort, determination, and willpower. But it does not require bouts of exhausting, strenuous exercise, nor joining a gym or using expensive equipment.

Formal and informal exercise

Fitting exercise into a busy routine can be difficult, but if you consider it a burdensome chore you will never do it. Exercise doesn't have to be "formal", in which you change into a special outfit, complete the exercise or activity, then return to normal life. Most activities that you do as part of your daily life are "informal" and therefore have the same potential health benefits as formal exercise.

Walking is a very good example of a simple but effective informal exercise or physical activity that is easy to do on your own without specialist equipment or facilities. Even gardening, shopping, doing the housework, or taking a day out can be seen as informal exercise or a physical activity.

More formal exercise activities, such as cycling, swimming, and exercise classes in a community centre, are very good of course, but they require extra effort, equipment, facilities, or sometimes supervision. In reality, you can exercise wherever you like, at home alone or with an exercise class – it makes no difference.

The important thing is to find an activity that you want to do – one that is enjoyable, affordable, and available. You also need to feel comfortable doing it. If you don't, you will probably soon stop. If you do feel comfortable, find the exercise level that is right for you and aim to maintain it.

PRACTICAL TIPS

EXERCISE ADVICE

Remember the following tips when you exercise:

● Always ensure you are stable and safe.

● Start a new exercise slowly and cautiously. Gradually increase the duration, frequency, and intensity of the exercise.

● Decide what you will do and when, where, and for how long you will do it.

● Set a realistic, achievable goal. When you reach it, set a more challenging, but still achievable, goal.

● If an exercise causes you prolonged pain, discomfort, or swelling, rest for a couple of days.

● Blood, sweat, and tears are not an essential – or desirable – part of exercise.

FORMAL EXERCISE
Exercising in the gym is a formal activity that requires special equipment and supervision to prevent you from damaging your joints and muscles.

Beginning to exercise

In general, people with arthritis should consult their doctor before embarking on a programme of exercise. Only a very few people should not exercise at all. These are very ill people with advanced, serious, and unstable medical conditions. If you are worried or need help, ask your doctor, physiotherapist, or nurse about what exercise you can do.

The vast majority of people with common stable conditions can begin exercising gently and build slowly without fear of adverse effects. Don't be too ambitious at the start. If you are not normally active, begin with gentle exercises that are not weight-bearing – for example, slowly bend and straighten your knees as you sit on a bed, sofa, or on the floor.

Over the following days, weeks, or even months, gradually increase the frequency and intensity of these exercises. Try to exercise for about 30 minutes on most days of the week. It doesn't have to be all at once – you could break it up into two 15-minute or three 10-minute periods.

Doing a little physical activity regularly is better than doing none at all. Within reason, the more you do the better. Remember, every little bit helps – you!

Your eventual aim is to practise weight-bearing exercises or activities that use your body weight as a resistance. Examples of these are stepping on and off a low step or standing up after sitting in a low

WALKING

Walking is probably the best and simplest way to encourage people with arthritis to be more mobile. However, they often find that walking increases their pain and this can be a worry.

- Make sure you are wearing good, supportive shoes or boots.
- If walking is painful, avoid long walks as they only make the pain worse. This will undermine your confidence and belief in your ability to help yourself.
- See how far you can walk before the pain starts and set a target well within this distance.
- Walk little and often within this distance at a comfortable pace.
- Rest if you need to. A walking stick may help you walk further.

- Gradually increase the amount you walk – walk rather than drive, get off a bus earlier, take a brisk walk around the block or park.
- Each week, increase the distance a little. Vary your walks to make them interesting, enjoyable, and purposeful. Go with friends, alternate walks to different places, take a day out, and visit local attractions.
- When the weather is too bad for you to go out, try to practise the exercises described on pp.160–171 indoors instead.
- If you do not walk regularly, start with a gentle short walk, well within your capabilities, at a speed and over distances that do not cause or increase severe pain. The next time you walk, go a little further or a little more briskly.

WALKING THE DOG
One way to encourage you to exercise is to walk a dog regularly. Make sure your joints can put up with the enthusiasm of a dog on a lead.

WALKING
For people with arthritis, walking is one of the best and most pleasurable ways to exercise. Walking is not too stressful or exhausting – simply walk regularly and comfortably at your own chosen pace.

chair (see p.166 and p.169). You can also begin with low-impact activities that do not cause pain, such as a gentle walk.

Whatever exercise or activity you do, be sure to pace yourself, balancing the activity with rest, without letting the reason for resting on painful days become the excuse for being inactive on relatively pain-free days.

Stretch yourself a little

Whatever exercise you do, try to exercise near to your maximum ability. This doesn't mean go all out and completely exhaust yourself. Rather, try to stretch yourself just that little bit more to get the best out of the exercise.

When you exercise you should feel slightly warm with your heart beating a little faster, but still able to hold a conversation – if you can't you're probably working a little too hard. How well you do an exercise is as important as how many repetitions you do.

GET ACTIVE
Joining an exercise class in your local community encourages you to get active and share the health benefits with others.

When you start any unusual activity, you will feel some aches or pains either during or after. If you experience increased pain or swollen joints for two to three days, rest for a few days until the pain subsides, then start exercising gently at a comfortable level.

Keeping going

You are likely to experience times when you cannot exercise because of pain, or because you're too busy, too tired, or the weather is bad. Accept this as inevitable but try to identify your potential barriers to exercise and plan ways to overcome them. Lack of time, pain, or bad weather may in fact be the reason you cannot exercise, but you may be tempted to use it as an excuse. Recognize this as a barrier and find ways to motivate yourself (see Motivation, left).

If your joints are painful, then rest for a while. If the weather is bad, leave exercising for a day. But then start again. Unless the pain is very bad you can still keep going and exercise gently within your comfort zone. If the weather is bad try to exercise indoors. The important thing is to resume exercising when the pain subsides, your enthusiasm returns, or the weather cheers up. Remember the importance of physical activity in maintaining your health – and keep motivated.

GOAL SETTING AND ACTION PLANS

Consider your current level of activity and the impact arthritis is having on your daily life. Ask yourself what activities you would like to perform more easily if you could. You can use these as goals that exercise and physical activity can help you achieve.

• Initially, set yourself simple, challenging, but realistic goals that you can achieve within a few days or a week – and pursue them in a very focused way. They should be important to you. People with arthritis often have great difficulty performing the common activities of daily living, but being able to do them more easily can have a great impact on a person's independence, personal satisfaction, and quality of life.

• Decide exactly what you are going to do – and when, where, and how you are going to do it. Be very specific to avoid making loose plans that tend to be put off and forgotten. Write this out in a formal action plan, pin it up on the wall where you can see it every day – and stick to it. After a while exercising will become a habit.

• Tell your family, friends, and colleagues about your plan. A public "declaration" can help you carry out your determination to exercise. More importantly, they can remind you to do things and can become a tremendous

REALISTIC GOALS
Set yourself a realistic goal that is achievable, given your current level of fitness. Not everyone will be able to jog along a pavement.

source of encouragement, support, and motivation.

• Monitor your progress. Circle on a calendar the days when you have exercised – and aim to cover it with circles. When you have achieved a goal, reward yourself with something you like. Appreciate how much you have improved. Tell people of your achievements – the encouragement they can give you may help to keep you motivated.

• If you want, revise your goals by making those you have achieved slightly more challenging so that you are always pushing the boundaries of what you do. With a little more effort you will be amazed at how much more you can do for yourself, how much easier life becomes and how much better you will feel about yourself.

• If you can't achieve a goal, don't worry about it. Reassess the goal and aim for something less ambitious and slightly easier, so you don't become disillusioned and undermine your belief in your ability to achieve what you want to achieve.

REACHING A GOAL
When you eventually reach the goal you set yourself at the beginning of your exercise plan, you will find you have achieved a level of fitness that you did not think possible.

Treating arthritis

For people with arthritis the prospects of good and effective treatment are better than ever. There is no cure for many types of arthritis, but healthcare professionals can help you manage your condition so you can live life to the full.

Finding the right medication depends on the type of arthritis you have, as well as its severity and impact on your life. Many drugs can help relieve pain, inflammation, or swelling, although deciding which is best may depend on your response to particular treatments.

Surgical treatments offer a safe, reliable option when drugs are no longer effective. Replacing joints, in particular the hip and knee, bring hope and an astonishing increase to the quality of people's lives, as they rediscover the joys of pain-free movement.

Easing pain, encouraging sleep, reducing fatigue, improving posture – these are the sorts of benefit that complementary therapies can bring. If you want to try these treatments, look into them carefully and preferably with the help of your doctor. You may find they offer valuable relief from symptoms of arthritis, especially when used alongside conventional treatments.

Drug treatment

Over the last half-century pharmacologists have tried increasingly to match specific drug treatments to particular diseases. They no longer seek a magic bullet to combat all the different types of arthritis and related musculoskeletal disorders. The treatment for gout, for example, is quite specific and different from the treatment for osteoarthritis, for which only less specific remedies exist. In most cases of arthritis, drug treatment is used in combination with other methods, such as physiotherapy. The following pages explore the range of drug treatments and highlights the potent and specific drugs available for rheumatoid arthritis.

Your doctor should be able to present both the advantages and disadvantages of drug treatment, allowing you to make your own informed decision.

Starting medication

Most people with arthritis need to start taking medication at some stage. Yet drugs are never the only treatment – rest and wearing a splint for a short time can help, too, while physiotherapy exercises may strengthen muscles around an affected joint. These steps are important because you want to avoid taking drugs if you can – no drug is totally free of side-effects.

You can buy a small number of drugs over the counter, taking advice from the pharmacist who sells them. For most, however, you will need to consult your GP, who may prescribe analgesics and non-steroidal anti-inflammatory drugs (NSAIDs) in the early stages of many types of arthritis. For more drug therapy that may be more potent, your doctor will normally refer you to a rheumatologist in a local hospital for expert advice.

In this way, your treatment proceeds in a stepwise fashion, moving from the simple drugs to the more complicated, which may be given either alone or even in combination, according to the severity of your disease. Often, the most potent drugs will be the most expensive, so cost needs to be considered as well.

Side-effects of drugs

If you are faced with the prospect of drug treatment it is only natural you should be concerned with knowing its side-effects. But don't forget the benefit you are likely to receive from the drug. Your doctor should be able to present both the advantages and disadvantages of drug treatment, allowing you to make your own informed decision.

In this chapter, side-effects will be mentioned only when they are severe; generic rather than trade names for drugs will be used. Sometimes people fail to realize that the composition of a drug remains the same, even though it is made by several manufacturers and has different trade names.

Drug interactions

The potential for an arthritis drug to interact with a drug used for another medical condition is vast. Several hundred drugs might be used for arthritis and many thousands of drugs that could theoretically be prescribed for other medical conditions.

Your doctor has access to full lists of drug interactions through guides such as the *British National Formulary* and so will be able to draw your attention to the most serious interactions of a drug.

Doctors who prescribe drugs, such as anticoagulants, which are notorious for interaction, will also provide you with whatever warnings you need.

By law, detailed specification of a drug's interactions must be given in the packet. You can also look on the internet or ask a pharmacist for advice, but do not rely wholly on either source to make a balanced decision.

Always ask your doctor about weighing the dangers against the benefits – you may find the benefits of a drug outweigh the chances of a risky interaction.

Analgesics

The simplest analgesic, available in most countries over the counter, is paracetamol. This painkiller can safely be taken in a dose of 500mg up to eight times a day (normally as two tablets four times a day as required) without any risk of

YOUR PHARMACIST
A pharmacist will know about the drugs you have been prescribed and may help to answer your questions about taking them.

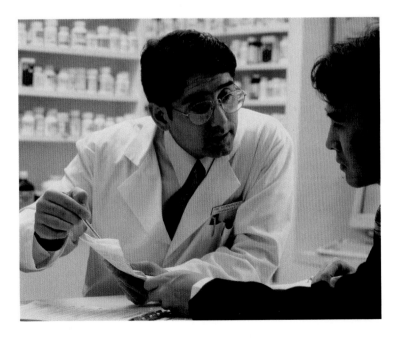

major side-effects. Avoid higher doses as they cause liver damage.

Paracetamol alone will relieve the pain of many types of arthritis. If it fails to do so and your doctor confirms the type of arthritis you have is a degenerative condition, which is less likely to respond to NSAIDs, your choice is to move to more potent tablets, such as co-codamol or co-dydramol. If these fail to help, your doctor could consider more expensive and potent analgesics – meptazinol or tramadol, possibly in that order.

Drugs remain under constant review by the licensing agencies in most countries. For example, in 2005, co-proxamol, arguably the favourite among the various analgesics for arthritis, was deemed unsafe. It was argued that the particular combination in co-proxamol was more potent than

co-codamol and co-dydramol in causing death if an overdose was taken deliberately. Many people with arthritis who dosed sensibly had already found co-proxamol to be particularly helpful. Currently, it is available on prescription on a "named basis" from a doctor.

NSAIDs

NSAIDs (non-steroidal anti-inflammatory drugs) are widely prescribed because they help people with many different types of arthritis, particularly types with an inflammatory component and where the joints are swollen, stiff, and sometimes a little hot, rather than just painful.

In early arthritis, you will normally be prescribed NSAIDs after you have tried analgesics.

TAKING DRUGS
Drugs for arthritis are normally taken by mouth, although they can be applied to the skin or injected, which is necessary if the stomach breaks down the drug.

NSAIDs have more side-effects than analgesics, although people who need them find them extremely effective. Only one NSAID – ibuprofen – is available over the counter and this is in a lower dose than that normally prescribed by practitioners.

Choosing the best NSAID

There are up to 40 or 50 NSAIDs marketed at present. You and your GP may wish to consider three factors when choosing the best NSAID for you.

First, the family to which an NSAID belongs has some bearing on the side-effects you are likely to experience. Some side-effects, notably gastrointestinal irritation, are common throughout the whole group so consult your doctor about protecting against them. Most NSAIDs also probably cause a slight but reversible change in kidney function.

Second, the length of time an NSAID lasts when a single tablet is taken is important. Some tablets need to be taken four or five times a day, others just once a day.

Third, the way an NSAID works on the inflammation process may be important. Usually, an NSAID blocks the action of a particular chemical in the body, known as an inflammatory mediator.

Of course, it is also important that you and your doctor decide which NSAIDs can help you to manage your pain cycle.

Q&A

Could I avoid the gastric side-effects by taking NSAIDs as a suppository?

No, not really. Many gastric side-effects actually result from the breakdown products of the drugs circulating in the blood rather than irritation of the stomach. Using suppositories as a route of delivery only reduces the risk slightly.

Cost concerns

If the cost of a drug is a concern, your doctor is likely to start prescribing from a list of older generic NSAIDs, which are long established as safe drugs.

The choice would be between short-acting drugs, such as ibuprofen and ketoprofen, that need to be taken four or more times a day; drugs, such as diclofenac and naproxen, that need to be taken two or three times a day; and drugs, such as piroxicam, that need to be taken once a day.

If none of these drugs suits you particularly and frequent dosing is found to be inconvenient, slow-release preparations of the shorter-acting drugs are also available.

COX-2 inhibitors

NSAIDs cause stomach problems because they block the action of a protective enzyme called COX-1. For this reason they are sometimes called COX-1 inhibitors.

A relatively new type of NSAID, called COX-2 inhibitors, is more specific and successful in suppressing inflammation, while at the same time protecting the gastrointestinal tract, particularly compared to the older drugs.

Experience from several years of prescribing COX-2 inhibitors has shown that they could predispose people to diseases of the heart and circulation. However, this is quite rare and many feel that if everyone on COX-2 inhibitors returned to the earlier drugs that cause gastric damage, the overall death rate would far exceed the death rate from cardiovascular side-effects.

It has been suggested that the risk of even a mild stroke or heart attack will only occur roughly once every 400 patient years of treatment and perhaps less often. Moreover, there is some evidence to suggest there is no risk if the drug is taken for less than a year.

The COX-2 inhibitors rofecoxib and valdecoxib were withdrawn in 2004 and 2005 respectively; celecoxib and etoricoxib remain; and lumiracoxib may yet be introduced. Following a review in 2005 by the EMEA (European Medicines Agency), doctors were advised to prescribe the lowest effective dose for the shortest possible duration.

You should discuss the risks of taking a COX-2 inhibitor with your doctor. A family history of heart disease or stroke would not necessarily prevent their use, but if you have previously had one of these conditions, seek medical advice. Alternatively, your doctor may advise you to return to an NSAID, with a second drug added to protect your stomach.

TOPICAL DRUGS
Some people enjoy applying cream to the affected area because they feel that they are actively doing something to help. Others find them messy and would be happy with a reduced dose of tablets.

Topical agents

You can buy NSAIDs, analgesics, and homeopathic remedies as a cream or paste for applying to the skin around your affected joints. These topical agents are absorbed through the skin more slowly than when taken by mouth. Therefore, side-effects are reduced but by no means completely avoided.

Little evidence indicates that topical agents remain in the joint for any significant period of time before they are taken away by the circulation. So topical applications may work in part by suggestion.

Counter-irritants, such as capsaicin (see p.116), are administered only by the topical route on the skin. The manufacturers of capsaicin point out that the only side-effect is pain at the point of application, but people soon acclimatize to this while perhaps forgetting the pain arising from the joint.

Steroid therapy

Treating arthritis with steroids has aroused much controversy among rheumatologists. Steroids are supremely effective in suppressing inflammation, but are responsible for a wide range of side-effects that detracts significantly from their use. These side-effects include suppression of the adrenal glands, high blood pressure, peptic ulcers, cataracts, and osteoporosis. In the various forms of arthritis, steroid use makes collagen fragile, which causes the skin to become fragile, too, and easily bruised.

Steroid use in early rheumatoid arthritis also remains controversial. There is a stronger rationale for using steroids when the disease is accompanied by inflammation of the arteries. For some conditions, such as polymyalgia rheumatica and giant cell arteritis (see p.34), steroids are very effective. There is also reasonable evidence for prescribing a small daily oral dose of steroids in rheumatoid arthritis of the elderly.

Intra-articular injections

Drugs injected directly into the affected joint – a technique called intra-articular injections – may be successful for many types of arthritis. The drug normally given is a steroid, which is particularly helpful when the inflammatory arthritis occurs at a single joint. One way to reduce the risks of the side-effects of the steroids is for your doctor to select, from the variety of steroid preparations available, a steroid that is relatively insoluble: it is more likely to remain in the joint for a longer period of time.

A wide variety of lubricants, such as hyaluronic acid, have been developed for use in intra-articular injection. These lubricants tend to be more expensive than steroids but their use may be more rational if your condition does not have an inflammatory component. Lubricants therefore tend to be used to alleviate the symptoms of osteoarthritis, which they often do for a short period of time.

Treating osteoarthritis

Preventive medicine involving exercise to strengthen the muscles around an affected joint is particularly important in the early stages of osteoarthritis. Some have favoured using specific local measures, such as taping the knee cap in osteoarthritis of the knee, as

Steroids are supremely effective in suppressing inflammation but carry a wide range of side-effects that detracts from their use.

NSAID TREATMENT OF OSTEOARTHRITIS

Weight-bearing joints such as the hip are particularly prone to the cartilage damage that is a feature of osteoarthritis. NSAIDs are commonly used to treat the pain and stiffness that accompanies the condition by reducing the inflammation in the joint. NSAIDs do not cure the disease, nor do they halt its progress.

Damage to the cartilage and bone tissue is followed by a response from the body's immune system and the release of chemicals called prostaglandins, which cause inflammation and pain. By stopping the production of these prostaglandins NSAIDs are able to reduce the inflammation in the joint and alleviate the pain.

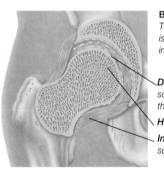

BEFORE TREATMENT
The cartilage in an osteoarthritic hip is damaged and the joint tissue is inflamed (left).

Damaged cartilage *in the hip socket and on the head of the thigh bone.*

Head of thigh bone

Inflamed soft tissue *surrounding the joint.*

AFTER TREATMENT
NSAID treatment reduces inflammation (right) and so helps to relieve pain but only for as long as the drug is administered.

Pelvis

The NSAID *reaches the tissues around the joint, where it stops the production of prostaglandins.*

Head of thigh bone

Reduced inflammation *in the soft tissues surrounding the joint.*

a means of delaying the start of symptoms or at least reducing them. Rest can often help, too.

Once these measures have been tried, your doctor will probably start you off with analgesics and then move to NSAIDs if analgesics alone fail to help or if there are inflammatory episodes with your particular type of osteoarthritis.

Often, the pain occurs only when you exercise, perhaps at a particular predictable time of day, such as when you walk out to do your shopping. In this case a drug of short half-life, taken just before you need it, is a more sensible approach than dosing yourself throughout the whole 24 hours.

Intra-articular injections and topical counter-irritants often help, too. However, if exercise suggests that your osteoarthritis is rapidly deteriorating at a small number of joints, you would normally be a candidate for surgery (which is very successful in this condition) before damage at one joint puts strain on others and the problem becomes more widespread.

Treating rheumatoid arthritis

More serious than osteoarthritis though less common, rheumatoid arthritis is an inflammatory condition that initially involves a joint and the tendons and tendon sheaths around the joint. As the disease progresses, however, it can involve other parts of the body, such as the eye, heart, lungs, skin, and blood vessels.

Many decades of research have led to the development of extremely potent and specific drugs; therefore, the management of rheumatoid arthritis is best based in hospitals. Some have "early arthritis" clinics: there is some evidence to indicate that if your rheumatoid arthritis is treated aggressively within the first 6 months, it is much less severe, although it would perhaps be over-optimistic to suggest that it could be cured.

In the very early days of your condition, analgesics are unlikely to be effective but NSAIDs may provide you with some relief. This may give you a false sense of security because the NSAIDs mask the symptoms but do not prevent progressive joint damage.

Such damage is best prevented by disease-modifying anti-rheumatoid drugs (DMARDs), which were specifically developed for this condition (though some of the earlier ones were discovered by chance). DMARDs represent the most specific type of drug and can be compared to fitting a specific key into the lock of a particular disease. Various DMARDs are available: tried and tested, and relatively inexpensive, they may be used alone or in combination (see p.87).

If your response to DMARDs is inadequate, you may be considered for a new generation of drugs called biologic agents. Developed since the mid-1990s, biologic agents specifically block the chemical messenger that causes rheumatoid arthritis in the early stages. Four are now available in the UK – infliximab, etanercept, adaminulab, and anakinra. More are likely to follow in the next decade.

One deterrent to prescribing biologic drugs is the expense – a biologic agent would be more than 15 times the cost of an older generation DMARD in standard dose. The financial implications have caused anguish in the health service, which has finite resources. With local individual trusts now given considerable autonomy by the government, decisions on funding are invariably local and so the chances of receiving biologic agents are higher in some parts of the UK than in others.

DMARDs

The following DMARDs may be prescribed in the treatment of rheumatoid arthritis:

■ **INJECTABLE GOLD** Introduced erroneously to medicine as a possible cure for tuberculosis, gold injections were found by chance to stabilize rheumatoid arthritis. Side-effects include skin rash, kidney damage, and depression of the bone marrow for which regular

Many decades of research have led to the development of extremely potent and specific drugs; therefore, the management of rheumatoid arthritis is best based in hospitals.

Since the start of the 1990s, most rheumatologists have regarded methotrexate as the most effective treatment for rheumatoid arthritis.

blood and urine checks are required. In spite of this, the drug remains remarkably effective in many individuals and is probably undervalued. An oral gold preparation (auranofin) was subsequently developed – it is less effective and often causes diarrhoea so it is rarely used.

■ **HYDROXYCHLOROQUINE** Anti-malarial drugs were also found by chance to improve rheumatoid arthritis. Several are available but hydroxychloroquine, although the most expensive, is probably the safest. A very rare but important side-effect is deterioration in vision for which regular eye checks performed by the prescribing doctor are advised. Otherwise, the drug is relatively safe though of only modest efficacy.

■ **AZATHIOPRINE** This prototype of a group of drugs developed against cancer prevents multiplication of cells. As rheumatoid arthritis is essentially a disease in which the synovium proliferates, it was realized that low doses would be effective in the management of this condition.

Side-effects include skin rash, liver damage, and depression of the bone marrow, for which regular blood checks are required. The drug has largely been replaced by methotrexate (see right).

■ **D-PENICILLAMINE** Although this drug was initially developed for rare metabolic diseases, it was noted that it reduced rheumatoid

factor in the blood. Trials showed it to be effective in giving partial control of rheumatoid arthritis.

D-penicillamine is probably less effective than injectable gold and, with the arrival of newer drugs, has become somewhat old-fashioned. Side-effects are skin rash, kidney problems, and bone marrow depression, for which regular blood and urine tests are required.

■ **SULPHASALAZINE** Developed for use in rheumatoid arthritis almost 50 years ago, this drug fell into disrepute and was taken over by gastroenterologists because it was effective in the treatment of ulcerative colitis and Crohn's disease. It was re-evaluated for rheumatoid arthritis in the early 1980s and proved to be effective after all. Invented in Sweden, it enjoyed European popularity at a time when methotrexate was being championed in the US.

Sulphasalazine is widely used and, although it shares some side-effects with methotrexate (such as damage to the bone marrow and liver, and skin rash), many feel they are not as severe. Regular blood checks are required.

■ **METHOTREXATE** Developed as a anti-cancer drug, methotrexate is very effective for psoriasis at doses much lower than those used in the treatment of cancer. In some people it sends psoriasis into remission. It is also effective for the arthritis associated with psoriasis. Trials subsequently found methotrexate to be effective in the closely related rheumatoid arthritis.

Since the start of the 1990s, most rheumatologists have regarded methotrexate as the most effective treatment for rheumatoid arthritis. Dosage is calculated according to your needs but it normally averages at 20mg a week. Some prefer intramuscular injection, which is often tried if the tablets prove unsuccessful.

Regular blood tests are required to guard against methotrexate accumulating in toxic amounts in the bone marrow and the liver. The drug can cause mouth ulcers and a rare but severe inflammation of the lungs. To guard against side-effects, folic acid is prescribed alongside methotrexate.

■ **CYCLOSPORIN** Developed from a fungus specifically to prevent rejection of kidney transplants, cyclosporin was found to have some action in rheumatoid arthritis. Arguably much less effective than methotrexate or some other drugs, cyclosporin is now used less frequently. Side-effects, which include increased blood pressure and impairment of the function of the kidneys, tend not to be severe, although they should still be monitored.

■ **LEFLUNOMIDE** Introduced in the mid-1990s, this drug is specifically designed for treating rheumatoid arthritis. It blocks one particular pathway in cell multiplication, arresting the spread of the disease.

It has proved remarkably effective in certain individuals and, in many cases, it now provides a second choice after methotrexate. Side-effects of leflunomide are raised blood pressure, an increased propensity to chest infection, and, sometimes, weight loss. On the whole, these side-effects are uncommon and not too serious.

Biologic agents

In the 1990s, scientists found that rheumatoid arthritis is switched on in the body by a chemical messenger called a cytokine, which is known as TNF–alpha. They discovered that another cytokine, known as IL–1, plays a secondary role in triggering the disease. Medical researchers have since developed a group of drugs named biologic agents to block

Q&A

My husband and I are hoping to start a family. Will the DMARDs I'm taking affect the baby?

Yes, the DMARDs may cause your baby problems, particularly in the first 3 months of pregnancy. As a general rule, you will probably need to stop taking DMARDs for 3–6 months before you conceive. Talk with your doctor before becoming pregnant and find out about the risks. You may need to discuss an alternative regime of drugs to help you cope with your symptoms until you conceive. For some people, their pregnancy "quietens" their rheumatoid arthritis.

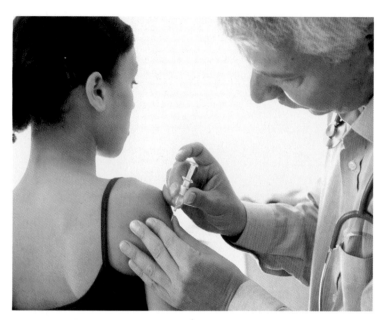

INJECTING DRUGS
Drugs may be administered by injections of different types. Nurses usually give injections under the skin or into the muscle, while doctors give injections directly into a vein.

though this remains under close review. A second theoretical risk that infections would be increased (since TNF–alpha protects against infection) has also not been substantiated, except for some chronic infections, notably tuberculosis where the risk is of awakening a previously dormant disease rather than catching the infection anew.

■ **INFLIXIMAB** This is an antibody against TNF–alpha. It is made partly in mice and so contains foreign mouse protein, which requires simultaneous methotrexate to be given in a low dose to prevent an allergic reaction. Infliximab has to be given intravenously, which often requires a half-day admission to hospital each time it is needed (usually every two months after two initial loading doses).

■ **ETANERCEPT** This competes with TNF–alpha in the body, displacing it from the places where it is harmful. In addition, etanercept can be used against some other cytokines. The drug is given by subcutaneous injection, normally twice a week.

■ **ADAMINULAB** This is an antibody that is made independently of animals and so is less likely to cause allergic side-effects. It is injected under the skin, normally every second week because it acts for longer than etanercept.

■ **ANAKINRA** This drug also needs to be given with a small dose of

and so neutralize these cytokines. They provide a much higher degree of disease specificity than the DMARDs.

Four such biologic agents are available: infliximab, etanercept, and adaminulab all block the action of TNF–alpha, while anakinra blocks IL–1. At present, all these drugs have to be injected.

The cytokines play such a fundamental role in regulating body disease that prescribing biologics has been cautious. The British Society for Rheumatology has established a national biologics register in the hope of detecting any adverse trends at the earliest possible stage.

To date, the theoretical anxiety that these drugs would increase susceptibility to cancer (since TNF–alpha protects against cancer) has not materialized,

methotrexate (see Infliximab).
It blocks the IL–1 cytokine but
its effects can be disappointing.

Combination therapy

The expense of biologic therapy
led rheumatologists to develop
specific combination therapies for
people with rheumatoid arthritis
who had tried some or all of the
available drugs. It is particularly
good for people who are newly
diagnosed with rheumatoid
arthritis. One combination uses
sulphasalazine, methotrexate,
and hydroxychloroquine.

The theory is that remission
from the disease is maintained
by the combination of drugs
acting on the body in different
ways, with less potent side-effects
because each drug is given at a
lower dose than if it had been
used on its own.

When prescribing a course of
combined drugs, a rheumatologist
usually reviews the many separate
DMARDs in turn, then proposes a
specific combination on the basis
of each person's idiosyncrasies.
In this way, a drug that was
previously discarded as ineffective
when administered alone might
prove effective when used in
combination with another.

Consequently, some people
with rheumatoid arthritis who
are denied biologic therapy on
the grounds of either availability
or high cost could be made quite
well with combination therapy.

TREATING OTHER TYPES OF ARTHRITIS

Osteoarthritis and rheumatoid arthritis are the most common types of the disease.
The drugs used to manage them often provide a starting point for doctors and
rheumatologists who are looking to treat other types of arthritis. For example,
DMARDs are used to treat ankylosing spondylitis and lupus, and analgesics and
anti-inflammatories are used for acute gout.

CONDITION	TREATMENT
Ankylosing spondylitis, psoriatic arthritis, and reactive arthritis	DMARDs such as methotrexate, azathioprine, and possibly leflunomide offer most promise. There is increasing evidence that biologic agents that block TNF–alpha are also effective. Injectable gold and cyclosporin are, at best, partially effective.
Lupus (systemic lupus erythematosus, or SLE)	The list of effective DMARDs is small. Hydroxychloroquine is particularly helpful and azathioprine is also used. If there is a severe accompanying vasculitis (see p.34), systemic steroid therapy with or without cyclophosphamide therapy may be required. Other biologic drugs are in development to block the cytokines relevant to lupus and its relatives.
Gout	Analgesics and anti-inflammatory agents have a role in managing acute attacks of gout. Long-term treatment is with drugs that alter uric acid metabolism. The most commonly used drug for this purpose is allopurinol.
Fibromyalgia	Antidepressants taken at night, in a dose much lower than that normally needed to relieve depression, significantly modify the symptoms of fibromyalgia during the day. The drug amitriptyline has been succeeded by dothiepin, and a variety of SSRI (selective serotonin re-uptake inhibitors) also display promise in treating this condition.

Surgical treatments

If one of your joints is damaged to the point where the pain cannot be controlled with drugs or the joint can barely move, then surgery may be the only answer. Modern surgical treatments that focus on specific joints are refined, safe, and usually successful. In fact, joint replacement surgery – particularly of the hip – has become one of the most effective treatments in the whole of medicine. Surgery offers longer-lasting solutions because surgeons now place additional emphasis on preparing people prior to their operation while other healthcare professionals focus on improving recovery and rehabilitation.

Operating theatres are equipped with ultraclean laminar airflow systems and dedicated wards help to maintain hygiene and reduce the risk of infection.

Candidates for surgery

The single most important sign that you might need surgery is the pain you continue to feel in one of your joints, despite the best efforts of other treatments. It does not matter which type of arthritis you have. For this reason, surgery may be a good option and your doctor may recommend it to you.

However, while surgery can address problems relating to an individual joint, an operation will not be able to stop arthritis that affects a number of joints.

How bad does your pain have to be before surgery is needed?

Two examples illustrate how the timing of surgery is crucial and why having surgery can be a difficult decision for you to make.

First, a retired woman who is in constant pain from an arthritic knee, especially pain that wakes her at night, would immediately benefit from a knee replacement and its likely 15-year lifetime.

Second, an active working man of 38 with an arthritic hip that hurts at the end of a long day would get pain relief from a hip replacement. However, although the implant would allow the man to remain active, the joint would need revising (see p.107) at least once, if not more, depending on the implant used. In other words, his operation needs to be repeated.

If you have arthritis, you and your surgeon need to weigh up the risks and benefits before making a decision about surgery. Advice from other health professionals and your family may be needed, too.

Who performs surgery?

Surgery for arthritis, and replacing joints in particular, is a highly specialized part of orthopaedic surgery. This branch of surgery has evolved from setting fractures in plaster to treating deformities of the skeleton, replacing joints, and dealing with complex trauma.

Many orthopaedic surgeons specialize solely in replacing joints, concentrating either on the hip, knee, or shoulder. Training for such a speciality can take a long time – often 10 years or more after qualifying as a doctor. Many large hospitals in the UK and elsewhere offer specialist fellowship training in joint replacement.

Joint replacement also requires specialist facilities and expertise in hospital. Operating theatres are equipped with ultraclean airflow systems and dedicated wards help to maintain hygiene and reduce the risk of infection.

Nursing staff are trained to care for the particular needs of people who are undergoing joint surgery.

Physiotherapists and occupational therapists are part of the multidisciplinary team working towards effective post-operative recovery and rehabilitation.

Surgical treatment options

Your orthopaedic surgeon has a number of treatment options to choose from, depending on the particular problem that affects your arthritic joint. Replacement of a joint is one of the most common procedures; others include washing out and fusion.

JOINT SURGERY

The main types of joint surgery available to orthopaedic surgeons include washing out, fusion, synovectomy, realignment, and total joint replacement. The chart below summarizes the purpose of each type.

TYPE OF SURGERY	PURPOSE
Washing out	To remove loose fragments from inside the joint.
Synovectomy	To remove the synovium from the joint.
Realignment	To correct a deformity or straighten a limb.
Fusion	To prevent joint movement.
Joint replacement	To replace all or part of a joint with an implant.
Spinal surgery	To relieve pressure on the spinal cord, to fuse adjacent vertebrae, or to remove an affected intervertebral disc.

Joint fusion is not common but it can still provide excellent pain relief in the wrist, big toe joint, and ankle by preventing the movement that causes pain.

Washing out

Bone and cartilage fragments can collect in a joint, such as a knee or elbow. They may be at least 1cm in diameter and can jam inside a joint, causing intense pain and loss of movement. Washing out the joint (see below), which has been practised for many years, especially on the knee, can relieve the symptoms.

The straightforward washing-out procedure may involve introducing an arthroscope (a fibre-optic tube with a microchip camera) into the joint, to provide a detailed view of the bone surfaces, cartilage, and ligaments. Instruments, such as forceps, remove the fragments and roughen the exposed bone on the surface of a joint (a process called chondroplasty) in order to stimulate new cartilage formation.

Some people experience relief of symptoms for a variable period of time, but there is no conclusive evidence that washing out and chondroplasty stop or slow the arthritic process.

Synovectomy

The synovium, or thin membrane lining, of a joint is the source of the chemicals that cause inflammation in rheumatoid arthritis and other types of inflammatory arthritis. Removing the synovium in a procedure called synovectomy may slow the overall process of your arthritis, although there is a risk of bleeding into the joint and post-operative stiffness.

Resection of a joint

In the past, one of the few effective surgical treatments for a painful joint was resection, which simply involved removing the joint. One example of this was resection of an infected hip joint. Few joints are treated this way today, although resection of the joint of the big toe, especially in elderly people, is still sometimes done.

WASHING OUT THE ELBOW

One surgical technique that is used to clean out fragments from the elbow joint is known as the "OK" procedure. Usually, an X-ray of the bone surfaces and cartilage of the elbow has revealed the presence of loose particles in the front of the joint. The surgeon makes a precise hole in the end of the bone in the upper arm (humerus) to provide suitable access to the front of the joint. It is important that this hole is sufficiently wide to allow the surgeon to insert instruments into the joint. Then the surgeon inserts a pair of forceps to carefully retrieve all the loose fragments of bone and cartilage.

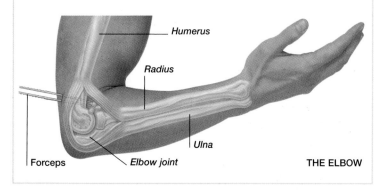

Humerus

Radius

Ulna

Forceps   Elbow joint   **THE ELBOW**

Joint realignment

Arthritis affecting certain joints of a limb may lead to a noticeable deformity. Surgical realignment of the joint (also called osteotomy) can, in some cases, reverse this deformity. The knee is the most common joint to be realigned in this way (see right), although the procedure can help in early disease of the hip joint, too.

Osteoarthritis of the knee mainly affects the inner part of the joint and may be associated with a bow-legged appearance of the legs. As the arthritis progresses, more load from the body's weight is transferred down through the inner part of the knee.

The procedure can often relieve pain and delay the progression of arthritis. However, it is only really suitable for relatively young people whose knee has a good range of movement and is not completely affected by osteoarthritis.

Fusion of a joint

Joint fusion, or arthrodesis, may seem an odd operation for arthritis, yet it has been widely performed in the past. Two examples are hip fusion after tuberculosis-related arthritis and knee fusion after post-traumatic arthritis.

At present, joint fusion is not common but it can still provide excellent pain relief in the wrist,

OSTEOTOMY OF THE KNEE

In the realignment, or osteotomy, of a knee the surgeon cuts through the shinbone (tibia) and wedges bone graft into the resulting incision. A metal plate is attached to the bone with screws to hold the incision open. The procedure straightens the leg so that the forces across the knee pass through the middle of the joint instead of the inner part. As a result, the load of the body on the knee is spread evenly across the whole of the joint. After surgery, the leg requires regular physiotherapy to keep the knee functioning until full fitness is restored – a rehabilitation process that takes between 3 and 6 months.

Thighbone

Kneecap

Bone graft
opens up the incision.

Metal plate
holds the incision open.

Screws
hold the bone in place.

Fibula

Shinbone

A REALIGNED KNEE
An osteotomy can realign the knee so that the leg remains vertical instead of leaning inwards.

big toe, and ankle by preventing the movement that causes pain. Problems occur because adjacent joints have to move more to compensate for the stiff, fused joint. If adjacent joints develop arthritis early, this extra movement can make them rapidly more painful.

Hip replacement is one of the most effective uses of healthcare resources. Over 45,000 total hip replacements are performed each year in the UK, and over 90 per cent are entirely successful.

To achieve a satisfactory fusion, the surgeon removes the affected joint surfaces and fixes the bone ends firmly together until the two have healed. The techniques of arthrodesis are similar to those of fracture healing – for example, the use of internal plates and screws.

Total joint replacement

Replacing joints, or arthroplasty, is the mainstay of surgical treatment for arthritis because artificial joints can provide many years of stable and pain-free movement. The success of total joint replacement is due to improvements in surgical techniques, the methods of fixing the implants in position, and the implants themselves.

Better manufacturing techniques and materials mean that implants rarely break yet can still move with minimal friction at the surface of the artificial joint.

Low friction was recognized as a key aspect of artificial joint design in the 1960s by Sir John Charnley, who is often regarded as the father of modern joint replacement.

Fixing implants

Joint replacement surgeons fix implants into position either with or without cement. Bone cement is a fast-setting polymer that binds the implant to the bone and transmits the load from the weight of the body between the two.

The polymer is applied as a viscous fluid to the bone, then pressurized to force it into the bone's porous surface. The implant is inserted and held motionless in position until the cement has set (approximately 10 minutes).

A cementless implant usually has a coating on its surface that encourages bone to grow into it and so achieve a more permanent fixation. Sometimes, the use of artificial bone substitutes, such as hydroxyapatite, can enhance this process. Once a cementless joint has been implanted, bone grows into its surface over a matter of months, firmly fixing it in place.

Hip replacement

If you are in constant pain, unable to move, and wholly dependent on others then a hip replacement can transform you into a pain-free, mobile, and independent person. Hip replacement has become one of the most effective treatments in the whole of medicine.

Early attempts to resurface the hip with metal moulds, or to insert sheets of tissue between the rough surfaces, were not usually effective. One surgeon even tried pig bladder as a cushioning layer, with predictable results!

Hip replacement is one of the most effective uses of healthcare resources. Over 45,000 total hip replacements (THR) are performed

TOTAL HIP REPLACEMENT

In a total hip replacement operation, the damaged ball-and-socket components of the hip are removed and replaced with artificial implants. The implants may be secured with or without cement (see opposite).

Removing the ball and preparing the socket

The surgeon makes a skin incision 10–25cm long and opens up the hip joint by carefully detaching the muscles at the top end of the thighbone (femur). The surgeon separates the ball (the head of the thighbone) from the socket and removes the diseased ball as well as the diseased cartilage lining the socket. He or she selects a metal cup to precisely fit into the socket and a very smooth inner plastic lining that fits into the cup.

The surgeon securely positions the cup to ensure the joint remains stable after the operation.

Inserting the artificial joint

The surgeon inserts the artificial stem into the thighbone and fits an artificial ball to the top. The ball may be made of metal, although more modern implants have ceramic balls that are much smoother and probably wear better in the long term. The surgeon places the new ball into the prepared socket, carefully re-attaches the muscles around the top end of the thighbone, and closes the skin.

ARTIFICIAL JOINT IN PLACE
An X-ray reveals a new hip implant in position, with the stem inside the thighbone and the ball sitting precisely in the plastic-lined metal cup.

ARTIFICIAL HIP JOINT

Pelvis

Pelvic socket An instrument called a reamer is used to remove damaged cartilage and bone from the hip socket.

Head of thighbone (femur) *has been replaced with an implant.*

Skin incision *is usually 10–25cm long.*

Shaft of thighbone *The centre of the thighbone shaft is hollowed out using a reaming device.*

Shoulder replacement

The operation to replace the shoulder joint has become very important for the treatment of arthritis and sometimes for the treatment of fractures around the shoulder joint itself. A half-joint replacement (hemi-arthroplasty) of the ball of the shoulder joint can produce good results.

The shoulder joint is a ball-and-socket joint much like the hip, although the socket is not so deep. Around the shoulder the rotator cuff muscles are very important in stabilizing the joint.

In rheumatoid arthritis, when these muscles are often in poor shape, a hemi-arthroplasty is usually effective for alleviating pain. The operation may not improve the shoulder's range of movement, but the joint should feel much more comfortable.

Total shoulder replacement is usually performed when the joint is affected by osteoarthritis. The success of the procedure often depends on how much bone is available in the socket, as this is usually the component that is most difficult to fix securely.

each year in the UK, and over 90 per cent are entirely successful.

In people over the age of 65, THR should have a 90 per cent or better chance of lasting 10 years or more, according to the UK's National Institute for Clinical Excellence. In practice, many well-established designs of THR last much longer than this.

Resurfacing a hip joint

The technique of resurfacing a hip joint is a modern and improved version of the implants that were popular in the 1960s and 1970s.

The surgeon mills the surface of the diseased ball and fits it with a metal cap, which is supported by a thin stem in the neck of the femur. The cap fits into a metal shell that lines the hip socket. People with a resurfaced hip often regain a very good range of safe movement. Whether resurfacing techniques will outlast conventional hip replacements remains to be seen.

Knee replacement

The introduction of new designs of implant that more closely simulate the structure of the natural knee has revolutionized

knee replacement over the past
15 years. Their predecessors were
often crude designs using a simple
hinge that did not allow the knee
its normal range of movement.
The modern total replacement is
an effective treatment for arthritis
of the knee (see right).

Modern knee designs perform
very well in alleviating pain. It
is possible their life span may
be greater than hip replacements.
The risks are very similar to those
for total hip replacement, so it is
important that you discuss these
with your surgeon before deciding
to have the operation.

Replacing part of the knee

Individual parts of the knee can be
replaced, too. The most common
operation is the unicompartmental
replacement of the inner side of
the knee. Such implants, which
replace only one part, can often
last 10 years or more.

Less common is the replacement
of the patello-femoral joint (the
joint between the kneecap and the
knee), although it is too early to
say how successful this procedure
will be in the long term.

Replacing other joints

Almost every joint in the body
can be replaced, although some
are more successful than others.
These include replacements of the
ankle, elbow, knuckles, and wrist.

TOTAL KNEE REPLACEMENT

The surgeon makes an incision down the front of the knee to open the joint, move the kneecap (patella) to one side, and expose the joint surfaces. The diseased cartilage is removed and cuts are precisely made in the bone to receive the metal replacements the surgeon has selected. These metal caps are very accurately positioned and attached to the top of the shinbone (tibia) – either with or without cement – and to the bottom of the thighbone (femur). The caps are shaped like the natural knee to allow free and easy movement. A plastic spacer placed in between keeps friction low and allows free movement without loosening the implant. The kneecap surface may also be replaced with a plastic insert.

REPLACING THE KNEE JOINT

KNEE IMPLANT
This X-ray shows a flexible knee implant that can bend like the joint it replaces. It is fixed into position with cement and attached by pegs into the bones.

Ankle replacement

Modern implants and improved surgical techniques mean that the replacement of the ankle joint is undergoing a renaissance, although historically it has not been particularly effective.

If rheumatoid arthritis affects your ankle, then you may well benefit from this procedure. One rare risk is that, in the event of the soft tissues around the ankle breaking down and infection developing, amputation below the knee may be necessary.

Elbow replacement

As a treatment for both arthritis and nasty fractures the replacement of the elbow joint is improving, although only a small number of surgeons perform this specialist procedure. If you have rheumatoid arthritis in the elbow it can bring significant improvements in your quality of life. It is rarely used for osteoarthritis of the elbow as this condition is relatively uncommon.

Wrist replacement

Replacement of the wrist joint is a very uncommon procedure and at present should be regarded as experimental. The technique may improve in the future, however.

Knuckle replacement

The replacement of one or more knuckles (metacarpophalangeal joints) is quite common in people with rheumatoid arthritis. These joints are sometimes replaced with silicone-like spacers that can give significant pain relief and improve the function of the hand.

Spinal surgery

All types of arthritis can affect the vertebrae of the spine. The spinal joints include the disc of cartilage (intervertebral disc) that cushions two adjacent vertebrae as well as the facet joints at the back of the spinal column.

Decompression

When osteoarthritis restricts the space for the spinal cord or the nerves emerging from it, spinal stenosis or lateral canal stenosis will result (see opposite).

Q&A

I have been offered minimally invasive surgery as a surgical option – what are the benefits and risks?

Minimally invasive surgery (MIS) reduces the size of incisions as a way of limiting blood loss and muscle damage during an operation. It may also speed recovery from joint replacement. However, there is some doubt about whether MIS for hip or knee replacement is as good as conventional methods. Risks include fractures of the thighbone and nerve injury. Find out how long your surgeon has been using MIS and what his or her success rate is.

If the stenosis is caused by bony spurs, the surgeon can widen the space in a procedure called decompression. This involves removing tiny chips of bone to relieve the pressure on the nerves.

If the stenosis is caused by the protrusion of a disc, the surgeon may perform a discectomy, which involves removing the protruding part of the disc.

Fusing vertebrae

Sometimes considerable pain can arise from an intervertebral disc that is diseased. Fusing the two adjacent vertebrae may relieve pain, but the outcome can be unpredictable and a failure of the fusion may lead to worse pain than was experienced before the operation. Vertebrae are fused by removing the diseased disc, then bone graft is used to stimulate the adjacent vertebrae to heal together. Nevertheless, if a particular intervertebral disc has degenerated yet the remainder of the vertebrae in the spinal column remains reasonably well preserved, then fusion can help reduce pain.

Disc replacement

Instead of fusion, a few surgeons have started developing disc replacements – some are based on metal and plastic, like those used in replacing a hip or knee. Disc replacement is at the experimental stage, as long-term results of this surgery are not yet available.

SPINAL STENOSIS

The spine is composed of many vertebrae, each with a space in the centre for the spinal cord to pass through. The spinal column is precisely stacked so that the spaces are perfectly aligned. If the space is reduced by bony spurs (osteophytes) or by the protrusion of an intervertebral disc, then pain will result. This narrowing is called spinal stenosis. Each vertebra is also designed to let the spinal nerves emerge from the cord. Narrowing of the spaces for these nerves is called lateral canal stenosis. If nerves to the legs are affected it often results in pain in the legs after walking a relatively short distance, although the pain can subsequently be relieved by sitting down.

NORMAL SPINAL CANAL
The precise structure of a vertebra means that the spinal cord has enough space to sit without restriction in the spinal canal.

Spinal canal

Spinal cord

Body of vertebra

Spinal nerve

Spinal canal *is reduced in diameter.*

DISC PROTRUSION
When a disc of cartilage that separates two vertebrae protrudes into the spinal canal, it can press on a nerve and cause pain.

Protruding disc *narrows the space of the spinal canal.*

Bony spurs *grow into the spinal canal.*

BONY SPURS
The bone of a vertebra may grow outwards and form spurs, or osteophytes. If these encroach on the space for the spinal cord or spinal nerves, they can pinch the nerves.

Body of vertebra

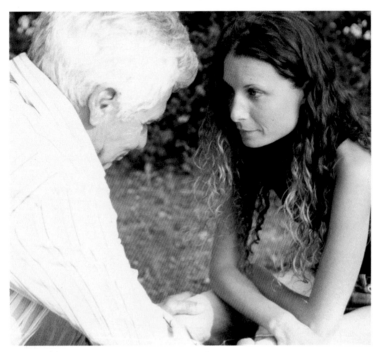

FAMILY SUPPORT
The encouragement and support of close members of the family can make preparing for hospital much less daunting.

Preparing for hospital

You should consider and resolve all kinds of issues and concerns before your surgery so that you are fully prepared for everything that surgery entails. This involves resolving medical problems so that you are fit for surgery, anticipating and organizing your work and care needs after surgery, making sure your finances are in order, and attending a pre-operative assessment clinic (see p.100).

Resolving medical problems

Most surgical procedures for arthritis are planned in advance (it is often called elective) so there is more than enough time to prepare thoroughly. Surgical success relies in no small part on careful pre-operative preparation, which identifies and treats potential problems, such as high blood pressure, diabetes, and asthma before a person's operation takes place (see p.100).

Efforts to reduce weight will improve general health, enhance the prospects of recovery from surgery, and may increase the lifespan of an artificial joint. The surgeon's life will also be made easier in the operating theatre.

Preparing for life after surgery

Before you undergo surgery, think about what life will be like after you have recovered. Discuss with your surgeon the restrictions you may need to impose on your work and lifestyle activities.

Find out what benefits you are entitled to and ask an occupational therapist what aids you may need. Talk to your employer before you plan time off for surgery, so they know well in advance about your potential absence – discuss your eligibility for sick pay and any modifications you may need when you return (see p.135).

■ **OFFICE WORK** Surgery may allow you to get back to work effectively if you have an office job that does not put too much pressure on your joints. You will probably be able to return to a sedentary job 6–8 weeks after surgery, but full function may not be achieved until 12 weeks has passed.

■ **HEAVY MANUAL WORK** If your job involves heavy lifting and carrying, talk to your employer about making modifications (see p.135) to reduce the reliance on your new joint. The heavy work involved in occupations such as building or farming place especially large loads on artificial joints and will reduce their lifespan as a result. It's a good idea to discuss your needs with an occupational therapist.

Arranging for care

Everybody who has surgery for arthritis will need some sort of help after the operation. Discuss your post-operative care in detail at the pre-operative assessment clinic (see p.100) so appropriate arrangements can be made.

For example, if you have a simple arthroscopic washout (see p.90), you will probably require help around the home for the first 24–48 hours, then you will need to be off work for about a week. Even young fit people, especially if they have more extensive surgery, will also require help, at least until they are able to recover from the tiredness they will inevitably feel.

Elderly people will require much more care after joint replacement surgery. Climbing stairs and steps as well as bathing and dressing may be difficult in the first few weeks. Family and friends may be able to help out, but social service input may also be necessary if no such help is available. In some circumstances a short period of convalescence in a suitable nursing home may be necessary after discharge from hospital.

Financial arrangements

If your surgery is done under the National Health Service (NHS) then you will not have to cover the cost of the operation or the hospital stay. Nevertheless, during the time you are in hospital, you may wish to arrange for paid help to look after your house and garden. You may also want the help to continue after you have been discharged.

If you wish to be treated privately, you can choose when you would like your surgery done, rather than having to spend time on an NHS waiting list. If you have private health insurance check well in advance of your surgery that your policy covers all the treatment costs, such as every aspect of your inpatient stay and outpatient consultations after you have been discharged.

If you can afford it you can pay for the surgery, but make sure you know exactly what your quote covers. Most quotes for fixed-price surgery include the fees for the surgeon and anaesthetist, all the inpatient costs, each test and investigation in hospital, and the physiotherapy until you leave. Some quotes do not cover the cost of subsequent outpatient consultations or physiotherapy.

PRACTICAL TIPS

GETTING FIT FOR SURGERY

● Take as much exercise as you can to improve your fitness and strengthen the muscles around your joints.

● If you have breathing problems, such as asthma, try to make sure your chest is as good as it can be. If you're a smoker, stop.

● If you are overweight, try to shed some extra pounds.

● Try to keep free from infections. This includes dealing with bad or loose teeth and infected toenails.

● If you are a woman on the contraceptive pill you may wish to stop taking it as it increases the risk of a blood clot. Find out more from your surgeon or doctor.

The pre-operative assessment clinic

It is very common for hip and knee operations to be performed under a spinal anaesthetic, so that you are numb from the waist down.

Make sure you attend the pre-operative assessment clinic as it is a vital part of the preparation for your surgery. Be prepared to stay for 3–4 hours. You will meet your surgeon and the pre-operative assessment team, which includes physiotherapists, nurses, and occupational therapists.

The assessment can highlight risk factors, such as high blood pressure, heart disease, and diabetes. By treating problems before surgery the team will reduce the risk of complications such as heart attacks, chest infections, and urinary infections.

■ **TESTS AND CHECKS** The team will take your detailed medical history, conduct routine blood tests, and may record an electrocardiograph (ECG) to check your heart. They may also take X-rays of your troublesome joint.

■ **INFECTIONS** Make sure you are clear of infection because it could spread to the treated joint. Infection in joint replacement surgery can be potentially very serious.

■ **REHABILITATION** A physiotherapist and an occupational therapist will talk to you about detailed aspects of your rehabilitation.

The occupational therapist will be particularly concerned that any modifications to your home are done before your discharge. For example, you may need handrails fitted beside your bath or shower or extra banisters installed on the stairs. If you are having a total hip or knee replacement, your seats and chairs – even toilet seats – at home may need to be raised before you return. The Disabled Living Foundation can advise you on equipment and aids (see Useful Addresses, p.215).

■ **BONE BANK** If you are having your hip replaced, you can donate the ball of your hip to the Bone Bank. It will be deep frozen and treated to eliminate infection, so that it can be used as a bone graft for people undergoing complicated revision surgery (see p.107), where they may have lost bone as a result of joints becoming loose.

If you agree to donate your bone, your blood will be tested for infections, such as HIV. However, you will be counselled thoroughly about the implications of this before you are tested.

Admission to hospital

When you are admitted to hospital for surgery, the admissions staff will take you to the appropriate ward and one of the ward nurses will check all your pre-admission details are correct.

Depending on the time of your admission, and the proposed time of your surgery, you should not have anything to eat or drink for 6 hours before the operation.

Q&A

What do I need to take with me when I go to hospital?

It is important to bring everything you need to make your stay in hospital as comfortable as possible. This includes dressing gown, nightwear, toiletries, plenty of reading material, and perhaps a personal CD player or radio. Make sure you bring several changes of clothing because you will be encouraged to get back into your everyday clothes as soon as possible after your surgery.

The consent form

Once you are comfortable on the ward, a member of the surgical team will visit you and mark the joint that needs surgery, as a fail-safe mechanism to avoid mistakes. The consent form, which you may have signed at the pre-operative assessment clinic, will be checked.

This form is very important because it records the discussion that you will have had with your surgeon and confirms that you are happy to undergo the procedure and understand the risks involved.

Anaesthetic techniques

Modern anaesthetic techniques allow joint surgery to be very comfortable, with very little post-operative sickness or nausea. You will have an opportunity to discuss with your anaesthetist exactly what technique is best for you, depending upon whether you want to be awake or not during the procedure, and taking into account any other medical factors or previous anaesthetic problems.

A traditional general anaesthetic is often used for joint replacement surgery, but may be supplemented by a local anaesthetic (which blocks nerve impulses) to numb the site of the operation.

Spinal anaesthetic

It is very common for hip and knee operations to be performed under a spinal anaesthetic so that you are numb from the waist down. This technique has the advantage of giving very effective post-operative pain relief, and you can choose either to be completely awake during the operation or to receive some sedation that allows

PRE-OPERATIVE TALK
Before you are due to go to the operating theatre, your surgeon will visit you. If there is anything more you need to know, now is the time to ask.

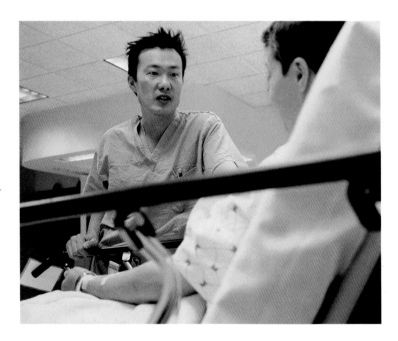

You should come round after the operation with little or no pain, and the recovery staff are there to ensure that your recovery is smooth and pain-free.

you to sleep. Many patients prefer the latter because they do not like to listen to the noise of the operating theatre.

Much upper limb surgery can also be performed under a local anaesthetic that blocks the nerves, with or without sedation or a general anaesthetic. A spinal anaesthetic can make passing urine after the operation difficult so you may need to have a catheter inserted into your bladder.

Avoiding blood transfusions

Surgeons and anaesthetists are constantly looking for ways to improve the safety of elective surgery. One particular area is the avoidance of blood transfusions wherever possible. A blood transfusion carries a very small risk of infection and can suppress the body's natural defence

Q&A

I would like to stay awake during my operation so that I can watch – is this a good idea and what sort of anaesthetic will I need?

Talk to your surgeon as well as other people who have watched their own operation before you make up your mind. Watching may make you feel nauseous and increase your anxiety. On the other hand, it may comfort you to feel a part of what is going on. You will be given a local anaesthetic so that only the area around the site of the operation becomes numb.

mechanisms. In other words, a blood transfusion might increase the chance of a post-operative infection. A healthy blood count at the pre-operative assessment clinic will reduce the need for a post-operative blood transfusion.

Saving blood lost at the time of the operation and returning it afterwards, particularly in knee replacements, may also reduce the need for a blood transfusion.

The day of surgery

When the time comes for your surgery, you will put on a gown and remove jewellery (except wedding rings), nail polish, and dentures. You may have a pre-medication to relax you. You will go from the ward to the operating theatre reception either in a wheelchair or on a trolley. You then go to the anaesthetic room outside the theatre where you will see your anaesthetist again and your surgeon will check you over just prior to the operation starting.

Coming round from surgery

When the operation is over you will return to the recovery ward either on your hospital bed or on a trolley. You will have an intravenous drip in one of your arms, and you may have drain tubes connected to drain bottles, which collect any blood lost after the operation. You should come

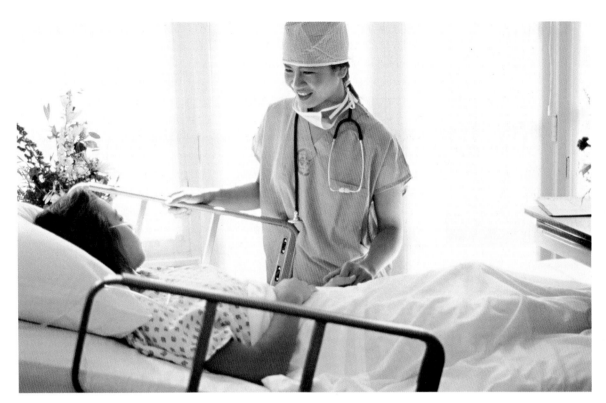

round after the operation with little or no pain, and the recovery staff are there to ensure that your recovery is smooth and pain-free. You will probably return to the ward within an hour or two of entering recovery, and later in the day you should be able to have short visits by friends or relatives.

Recovery in hospital

Drips and drains are usually removed within the first 24 hours after surgery, and you will be helped out of bed by the nursing staff or physiotherapists at this stage. If you have had an operation on your arm then physiotherapy

can start straight away, but if you have had an operation on your legs you will be gently mobilized with the physiotherapists to start with.

Recovery milestones

If you have had lower limb surgery the milestones you need to achieve in hospital include walking safely with crutches or a frame, getting into and out of bed, and getting into and out of a chair. The physiotherapists will check if you can negotiate stairs and steps.

Once you have passed all these milestones then it will be safe for you to go home. Some outpatient physiotherapy, especially after knee replacement, may be needed. If you have had a knee operation,

WAKING UP
After your operation you will probably feel tired and weak, but be reassured that ward staff are always present to monitor and help with your recovery.

GETTING BACK ON YOUR FEET
Physiotherapists will need to know you have reached all the recovery milestones before it is safe for you to go home.

the physiotherapists will be keen to see the muscles around the knee recovering and to know you have regained a good range of movement prior to your discharge.

At the time of discharge

Discharge planning is important to make sure the outcome of your operation is as good as possible. Dissolving stitches are often used, but if you have stitches (sutures) that need removing, plans for their removal will be made. Stitches can either be removed at your GP surgery or by a district nurse.

At the time of discharge checks will be made to ensure that all the necessary modifications to your home are in place, and that any social services care is ready for you when you get home. The hospital should also give you contact numbers to ring if you do have any problems after your discharge.

Rehabilitation milestones

When you get home from hospital you will probably feel very tired, no matter what type of operation you have had. Rehabilitation milestones will vary, however. For example, an arthroscopy on your knee will probably make walking uncomfortable for the first few days, but you should be able to return to work after perhaps a week or 10 days.

Milestones for total hip or knee replacements

A total hip replacement or total knee replacement will probably mean that you have to keep using your crutches for perhaps 4–6 weeks after the operation. This period may seem like a long time but it will give both your muscles and your wound a chance to heal nicely. You will then start coming off crutches gradually, perhaps on to a stick, but you should notice your level of mobility will be improving steadily.

Discuss with your surgeon when you can return to driving a car, although it is usual to wait perhaps 4–6 weeks after lower limb joint replacement surgery.

As long as you do not have many other joint problems, you will probably be off sticks and crutches completely by 10–12 weeks after the operation. At this stage you should be walking freely and really starting to get back to a normal life.

During recovery from lower limb joint replacement it is important to walk a little each day because this will help your recovery and also minimize swelling in your leg. You will be able to undertake short journeys in a car as a passenger almost immediately after discharge from hospital, but if any longer journeys are planned within the first 12 weeks after surgery, then you should stop regularly to get out and stretch your legs.

Complications during rehabilitation

A few complications can develop after any surgery and during rehabilitation, but the risks that are particular to the surgery of arthritis include infection, blood clots, and dislocation. There are a couple of rare complications, too.

Long-term monitoring and follow-up is important so that any problems that may develop with a replaced joint are identified early (see Revision Surgery, p.107).

Infection

In orthopaedic surgery, infection in an implant or bone can be very difficult to treat without further surgery. However, the risk of infection is not high – in total joint replacements, for example, it is about 1 in 200.

Surgeons make every effort to reduce the risk of infection during orthopaedic surgery. You receive antibiotics and your operation is performed in a special ultra-clean theatre by a team wearing special surgical suits.

After your operation, bacterial infections that form pus must be treated promptly to stop the germs spreading in your blood and attaching to the joint replacement.

However, if bacteria do enter a joint replacement, they can stick to the implant. At this stage antibiotics have no effect so the only way to eradicate the bacteria is to remove the infected implant, let the infection clear, then insert another new implant. This two-stage approach often requires 8–12 weeks between the two stages, and is obviously a major undertaking for the patient.

If you need significant dental work, ask your surgeon and dentist whether you should have a single dose of antibiotics first.

Blood clots

The risk of a blood clot (deep vein thrombosis, or DVT) developing in one of your legs is about 1 in 20, especially after an operation on your legs or pelvis. Reducing your weight before surgery, and getting mobile soon after surgery, can lower the risk. A blood-thinning agent such as heparin can help prevent blood clots, too. You may also be encouraged to wear special support stockings or intermittently inflating boots to prevent blood from pooling in your legs.

Q&A

How soon after my operation will I be able to fly?

It is probably not a good idea to fly until 12 weeks have passed after your surgery because of the slightly increased risks of blood clots (deep vein thrombosis). Many people notice that their joints continue to improve for at least 12 months after the operation, at which stage they almost forget that they have ever had the operation.

Q&A

If I take a blood-thinning agent such as heparin, what happens if I cut myself?

You should contact your doctor at once if you cut yourself or have a nosebleed or notice blood in your urine. Your doctor will probably prescribe a drug that helps your blood to clot.

The younger you are when you have your hip or knee replaced, the shorter time it is likely to last, as younger people use their joints more vigorously.

Blood clots can be treated and so do not usually lead to long-term problems. In some circumstances the blood clot can reach the lungs (a pulmonary embolism) and may be life-threatening.

Dislocation

If you have had a total hip replacement, there is a small risk that your new joint may dislocate, where the ball and socket of the new joint come apart. This risk, which is probably only 1 or 2 in 100, is highest in the first 6–12 weeks after your operation.

It is important to follow the advice of your physiotherapists and avoid getting your limb into a situation where dislocation may occur. Of course, you can use the joint, but respect it and avoid overloading it repeatedly or forcing it into awkward positions. If you have had a total hip replacement, don't cross your legs or bend over too far too soon.If you have had a knee replacement, don't kneel on it.

Rare complications

If you have surgery on a limb there is an extremely low risk of a nerve injury. Your surgeon will probably explain this to you at the pre-assessment clinic (see p.100).

Another rare complication is excessive bleeding after your joint replacement operation. This can result from an injury to a major blood vessel.

Long-term outcome

A replacement joint should last for many years, especially if you look after it. Studies of large numbers of people with joint replacements give statistical chances of how long a joint will last. For example, data from Sweden suggests that many hip replacements have a better than 80 per cent chance of lasting 20 years or more, before they need to be revised (see right).

The younger you are when you have your hip or knee replaced, the shorter time it is likely to last, as younger people use their joints more vigorously.

Knee replacement is now as good as replacement of a hip, and similar survivorship figures are reported. Upper limb joint replacements are obviously not placed under as much load as lower limb joints, which means that replacement shoulder and elbow joints may also last for many decades.

Revision surgery

If you have had a joint replaced and then it begins to fail, it is usually because the implant loosens inside the bone. The load-bearing surface of the implant also wears slowly. This is to be expected as a hip or knee may go through a million movements each year in normal use. As a result, you may be a candidate for revision surgery and a new joint.

An X-ray will enable your surgeon to detect what is wrong. As the joint loosens, it might become painful. Sometimes, a joint can loosen without pain and so you are unaware that the bone around your implant is becoming very thin. For this reason, your joint replacement should be X-rayed every 5 years or so, even if you feel absolutely fine.

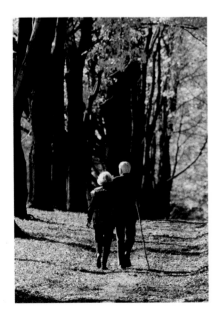

If your new joint loosens, you may need a revision. Surgical revision techniques have developed considerably and it is now possible to rebuild worn-out joints with new ones, using bone grafts to fill areas where the bone has become very thin or weak. A joint can be revised several times in theory – it all depends on how much bone is left after the old joint has been removed and how much scarring of the soft tissue has occurred.

Risks of revision

Revision surgery takes longer, is technically demanding, and is usually performed by specialists. Nevertheless, a successfully revised joint can perform almost as well as the first one, giving you back your mobility and independence.

The risks of revision surgery are higher than those for the primary operations. Candidates for revision are older than when they had their first operation and their general health may not be as good.

For each subsequent revision operation, the risks of infection go up. The muscles, ligaments, and skin become more scarred and fail to heal as well. Blood loss can be greater and surgeons rely more on saving blood cells (see p.102).

A BRIGHT FUTURE
Total joint replacements should last for a long time without causing any problems, allowing you to enjoy a bright future with plenty of activity.

Complementary therapy options

As well as exploring conventional treatments for your arthritis, you may decide to investigate some of the complementary therapies available now. Used wisely, these may help relieve certain symptoms, or simply contribute to your sense of wellbeing. You will find a great variety within the therapies. Some, such as herbal medicine, have been around for a long time, while others are relatively new. But the "complementary" part is key: the therapies complement, rather than replace, your regular treatment.

Since the mid-1990s, the market for complementary therapies has expanded at an unprecedented rate.

Therapies that treat the body and mind

Complementary therapies usually focus on treating the body and mind – in other words, the whole person. Practitioners of the therapies do not impose treatment but instead encourage healing to come from within the individual, who is an active participant. This holistic approach is based on the idea that health comes from a balance between the mind, body, and surrounding world. Any "imbalances" between these can result in poor health, low energy, or specific illnesses.

How therapies help

Pain is perhaps the primary symptom of arthritis and one of the most complex areas of human biology. We still do not know why some people experience more or less pain than others, although most doctors agree that state of mind can have an effect.

Some complementary therapies may simply help you to relax, reduce stress, or encourage sleep, which in turn may help to relieve pain. Side-effects are a common problem with some conventional drugs and this may prompt people to explore other ways of managing their condition.

The rise in popularity of the therapies

Since the mid-1990s, the market for complementary therapies has expanded at an unprecedented rate. The evidence for this can be seen in both the increased numbers of practitioners offering their services and in the enormous range of herbs and supplements that are available from health shops, supermarkets, chemists, and even corner shops.

But unlike the tightly controlled world of conventional medicine, it is a market that is largely without regulation and so safeguards for the public are not automatically in place. While doctors, for example, spend a number of years studying and gaining practical, supervised experience, practitioners of many complementary therapies do not necessarily do so and may freely start a business without any medical background or training.

A lack of hard evidence about the safety and effectiveness of many therapies means the medical profession remains sceptical about their validity. The good news is that universities and government bodies are spending an increasing amount of time and money on research into particular therapies. This should help to establish better evidence-based practices in the future and bring better safeguards into the practice of complementary therapies.

Controls on the sale of supplements

In an attempt to regulate the more unscrupulous parts of the health market, many countries are starting to control the sale and quality of herbs and supplements. Some of these have side-effects and potential interactions with certain medical drugs.

For example, a ruling from the European Court has placed some restrictions on the sale of certain supplements. As a result, around 200 varieties of supplement cannot be sold to the public and member states have until 2009 to stop their sale. All supplements for sale must appear on an approved list and those banned include tin, boron, and silicon.

The European Court also banned so-called "megadoses" of certain vitamins – supplements with many times the recommended daily amount (RDA).

Categories of therapy

Broadly speaking, the hundreds of different complementary therapies can be grouped into 3 categories: natural remedies and supplements, bodywork therapies, and movement therapies. However, this does not mean you can only try one therapy at a time. You can mix and match; for example, you can take a supplement and try a bodywork therapy.

MYTH OR TRUTH?

MYTH

If something is natural, it must be safe.

TRUTH

There are many dangerous substances within nature and natural remedies may still cause side-effects and have interactions with other drugs. As with any medicine, you must always follow the recommended dosage.

BODY MASSAGE
A professional massage can work wonders for easing aches and pains, relieving stress and improving your overall feeling of health and wellbeing.

"touch therapies", where a practitioner uses a hands-on approach to treatment. All involve work with one or more parts of the body, whether through manipulation (such as massage), touching techniques (such as reflexology), or use of implements (such as acupuncture). See pp.120–125 for more information.

■ **MOVEMENT THERAPIES** This group of therapies is based on learning to use your body to promote strength and wellness. Practitioners will teach you how to carry out the relevant exercises or movements. Usually, the therapies are not just systems of exercise but also use the mind to help facilitate bodily harmony. See pp.126–131 for more information.

■ **NATURAL REMEDIES AND SUPPLEMENTS**
Usually produced from substances found in nature, natural remedies and supplements are not yet as strictly controlled as conventional medicines. As a result, there may be a big difference between their quality, effectiveness. and safety.

Since certain supplements and herbs can sometimes interfere with the actions of drugs you may be taking, and because not all natural remedies are suitable for everyone, it is vital to choose reliable brands and to speak to your doctor before you try anything new. See pp.112–119 for more information.

■ **BODYWORK THERAPIES** This group encompasses those therapies that are sometimes referred to as

Finding a reputable practitioner

Many European countries require complementary practitioners to have a recognized medical qualification before they can practise their therapy or train someone else. This is not the case in the UK, where there are many excellent practitioners who are highly trained and professional, yet perhaps just as many who are not. For this reason it is important to choose a practitioner carefully.

Many of the more established complementary therapies have some self-regulation which is administered by their professional bodies. Practitioners who wish to be listed with a professional body must adhere to certain standards, such as completing a certified level of training. In return, the practitioner can be registered on an approved list, which you may be able to access online (see Looking Online, right).

Talking to your doctor about therapies

Although some doctors remain very sceptical about the integrity of complementary therapies and their place in the delivery of health care, an increasing number recognize their value, especially homeopathy and acupuncture.

Q&A

How much do complementary therapies cost?

The prices you may expect to pay depend on the practitioner, the therapy, where you live in the country, and whether you have a course of treatment or a one-off session. Your first introductory meeting is often the longest and most expensive session. Always ask at the beginning what the treatment will cost, whether any supplements or remedies are included in the price, and how many treatment sessions the therapist thinks you may need. Remember that complementary therapy for chronic diseases is not covered by private health insurance.

If you have heard that a specific therapy may be able to help your arthritis, the best first step is to talk to your doctor, who may be able to recommend an experienced practitioner in your locality. In fact, your doctor may even be the first to suggest a therapist as part of your treatment.

In the UK, many primary care trusts have their own particular access to services within the field of complementary medicine. A recent survey in the UK showed that 40 per cent of GP practices can now make such therapies available to their patients.

In addition, some doctors are themselves trained in a particular therapy, such as homeopathy or acupuncture. It is also common for hospital pain clinics (see p.47) to offer complementary health services to patients.

Keeping your doctor informed

If you are trying a complementary therapy, make sure you keep your doctor or rheumatologist informed. They can tell you if a particular herb or supplement is safe to take at the same time as any existing medication; they will also know whether a therapy suits your level of overall health and mobility. It may help you to take notes of any changes a therapy brings to your health, whether good or bad, which you can then discuss with your doctor.

PRACTICAL TIPS

LOOKING ONLINE

Many people turn to the internet and look online for information about health. Much of it is accurate, up to date, and useful, but some websites are unreliable. There is little or no regulation about health information on the internet. But there are ways you can stay safe:

● Check the credentials of the organization concerned. These should be clearly displayed on the website.

● Check whether the website has something called an Editorial Policy. Health sites should have both a Medical Editorial Policy and an Editorial Policy, which means that its content will be reviewed by other doctors.

● Be wary of advice that seems to contradict the information you have been given by your doctor.

● Be cautious of websites that are selling services or products. It is harder for such sites to be impartial about their advice.

Natural remedies and supplements

For thousands of years, people have turned to natural remedies to relieve their arthritis symptoms. The list of herbal medicines, supplements, and natural preparations seems to grow ever longer, with remarkable claims being made about their efficacy yet very little hard scientific evidence to back them up. A few, such as glucosamine, chondroitin, and omega-3 fatty acids, may genuinely help, while others seem to have no effect whatsoever – some may potentially interact with medication.

Chondroitin may be able to help with some aspects of joint health, such as lubrication, building cartilage, and making cartilage more elastic.

Common dietary supplements

People with arthritis are faced with a huge range of products that may or may not help their symptoms. Some supplements may only help certain kinds of arthritis. The choice of products, coupled with often conflicting stories in the press about their safety and their effectiveness, can make choosing a supplement daunting.

Glucosamine
An amino sugar found naturally in the body's cartilage, glucosamine may help with joint repair. Several studies have shown that it may be moderately beneficial for the pain and stiffness of osteoarthritis, particularly of the knee. Other studies suggest that it may be as effective as ibuprofen for pain relief, although the supplements needed to be taken for at least 2 weeks to have an effect.

Glucosamine supplements may be synthetic or include shellfish extracts. The recommended dosage is 750mg of glucosamine, taken twice a day. It is often combined with chondroitin (see right). This combination appears to help some people with moderate to severe knee pain due to osteoarthritis.

Glucosamine has no serious side-effects. Avoid it if you have an intolerance or allergy to shellfish, or if you are diabetic.

Chondroitin

This substance is found naturally in the body and is thought to protect cartilage and give it elasticity. Supplements are usually made from the windpipe of cows but do not carry any risk of BSE (a disease in cows that has been linked with a variant of Creutzfeldt–Jakob disease).

A large study of all available evidence has shown that chondroitin can help with some aspects of joint health, such as lubrication, building cartilage, and making cartilage more elastic. It may also reduce inflammation.

Chondroitin has no toxic side-effects so it may be worth a try. The recommended dosage is 600mg of chondroitin, taken twice a day. If you experience no benefits within 2–3 months, chondroitin probably does not work for you. If you take warfarin, or have a disorder that affects clotting, check with your doctor before taking chondroitin.

Fish oils

Oily fish, such as salmon, herring, mackerel, tuna, and halibut, as well as cod's liver, contain omega-3 fatty acids, such as EPA and DHA. These are important for brain function. More than 20 trials have shown that EPA and DHA inhibit the development of rheumatoid arthritis. They also help to boost treatments for depression and lower high blood pressure.

The recommended dose is as much as 3g of fish oil supplements a day, which may mean you have to take as many as 10 or even 15 capsules a day. You may experience certain side-effects such as nausea and nosebleeds. Do not take them with anticoagulants such as warfarin. Only take supplements that are labelled as being free of carcinogens, such as dioxins, that come from pollution in the sea.

Flaxseed oil

Flaxseeds contain an omega-3 fatty acid called alpha linolenic acid (ALA). The body may convert this into the fatty acid EPA, which has anti-inflammatory properties.

Although flaxseed oil appears to have many benefits, the scientific evidence has not yet confirmed

PRACTICAL TIPS

TAKING SUPPLEMENTS

- Before you take a product ask your doctor about its side-effects and potentially harmful interactions with other drugs.

- Only buy brands from reputable companies.

- Don't mix supplements – find out which ones help and which ones don't.

- Report any side-effects to your doctor.

- Always take the recommended dosage.

- If you're breastfeeding or pregnant, ask your doctor before taking a supplement.

- Never give supplements to children without first asking your doctor.

FLAX
Flax plants (*Linum usitatissimum*) are cultivated for both flaxseed oil and linseed oil.

that it relieves the symptoms of arthritis. However, people who do not want to take fish oils can try flax oil as an alternative.

Try flaxseed oil in capsule form or add it directly to your food – for example, as a salad dressing. It is a natural laxative. However, it may interfere with blood-thinning drugs, such as warfarin, and should be avoided by women with uterine cancer or hormone-sensitive types of breast cancer.

Collagen

Collagen is a protein found in the body's ligaments and connective tissue. Some scientific evidence suggests that Type II collagen, made from chicken breastbones, may help to relieve swollen and tender joints. Several studies suggest that undenatured collagen (collagen that has not been altered by heat) can help with the mobility and health of joints.

The recommended dosage of undenatured collagen is 60–500 micrograms a day. It has no known interactions with medications, but you should avoid it if you are allergic to chicken or eggs. Consult your doctor before trying any Type II collagen supplements.

Cetyl myristolate (CMO)

CMO is a type of fatty acid derived from beef tallow. It may help to relieve inflammatory conditions such as rheumatoid arthritis by acting on the immune response

involved. CMO is also said to help mobility by keeping joints supple. However, there is no strong evidence that CMO works, nor that it is either dangerous or safe.

Methylsulphonylmethane

This substance, also known as MSM, is found naturally in the body, as well as in fruits, grains, and vegetables. You can buy it as a supplement to take by mouth or as a gel or lotion to apply externally to affected joints.

MSM has been touted as a remedy for inflammation in arthritis, but there are no independent human studies to support this. It is not known exactly what effects MSM may have in the body. It may interfere with blood-thinning drugs, such as warfarin, and should not be used without informing your GP or rheumatologist first.

MSM was discovered as a by-product of dimethyl sulphoxide (DMSO), an unpleasant-smelling chemical that is said to relieve inflammation in joints and soft tissues if applied externally to the skin. However, it is not legally available as a supplement and can be highly toxic if it is poor quality. Do not take DMSO without your doctor's guidance.

Melatonin

This hormone is produced by the pineal gland in the brain and is involved in regulating the body's

Some evidence suggests that people with pain, morning stiffness, and joint tenderness may derive some benefit from GLA.

sleep–wake cycle. The level of melatonin in the blood is highest at night. It can also be found in some plants and foods. Melatonin supplements are usually synthetic, but some may be derived from animals. Although it is not used as a remedy for arthritis as such, melatonin may help the insomnia associated with chronic or acute pain, although the evidence for this is contradictory.

Do not take large amounts of melatonin supplements because there is evidence that doing so may be linked with depression. Melatonin may increase the effects of some of the drugs prescribed to combat anxiety.

S-adenosyl-L-methione

This substance, also known as SAM-e, occurs naturally in the body where it plays an important part in chemical reactions. It is claimed to help various conditions, including the pain and stiffness associated with arthritis, and fibromyalgia. Several trials show that SAM-e has pain-relieving and anti-inflammatory benefits.

SAM-e comes in tablet form or can be given as an injection. Many people tolerate it better than NSAIDs. High doses can cause gastrointestinal problems and headaches. Avoid SAM-e if you are taking monoamine oxidase inhibitors or antidepressants, or if you have a bipolar disorder or Parkinson's disease.

Gamma linolenic acid

This fatty acid, also known as GLA, is available as a supplement and also in the oils of borage and evening primrose. Oils containing GLA have been shown to reduce the inflammation in rheumatoid arthritis. Some evidence suggests that people with pain, morning stiffness, and joint tenderness may derive some benefit from GLA.

The recommended dosage is 1,800mg of GLA supplements a day. You will need to take considerably more borage oil or evening primrose oil to receive the same amount of GLA.

EVENING PRIMROSE
Evening primroses (*Oenothera biennis*) grow wild but are also cultivated for their oil, which contains GLA and has several beneficial properties.

Herbal medicines

Few herbs have been tested for their effect on the symptoms of arthritis, but evidence suggests that some may help relieve inflammation and pain.

Cat's claw

This vine (*Uncaria tomentosa*) grows in the Peruvian Amazon and has thorns shaped like a cat's claws. The root bark is a remedy for inflammation and has been used for boosting immunity, as well as treating arthritic and gastrointestinal complaints. Two studies suggest it may be useful for treating osteoarthritis and rheumatoid arthritis.

The recommended dosage is 500–1,000mg of cat's claw, taken as capsules three times a day. Medical herbalists often avoid using it with hormonal drugs, insulin, or vaccines because of potential interaction.

Devil's claw

This shrub grows in southern Africa and has hooked, claw-like seed pods. It contains a substance called harpagoside, which has been shown in two trials to reduce inflammation and pain. Devil's claw is a popular remedy among people with rheumatoid arthritis.

You can take devil's claw as a capsule or as a tincture or tea. It may interfere with warfarin or drugs used for irregular heartbeats and diabetes. Check with your doctor first if you have gallstones or gastric or duodenal ulcers. Avoid devil's claw if you are pregnant or are taking NSAIDs (see p.78).

Devil's claw is a popular remedy among people with rheumatoid arthritis.

DEVIL'S CLAW
The root of devil's claw (*Harpagophytum procumbens*) is a traditional remedy for relieving pain and inflammation.

Cayenne

Also known as paprika, chilli pepper, or red pepper, cayenne (*Capsicum frutescens*) is a remedy for various conditions, including arthritic pain and stomach upsets. Capsaicin, its active ingredient, stimulates the release of endorphins, the body's own pain relievers. Although there is little scientific evidence of its effectiveness, many people with arthritis regularly rub capsaicin cream into their affected joints.

You should avoid putting the cream on to broken or irritated skin. Wash your hands thoroughly after use. Eating too much cayenne can be highly dangerous as it affects your body temperature.

Boswellia

This herb (*Boswellia thurifera*), which produces the frankincense resin, is used in Chinese and Ayurvedic medicine for the relief of arthritic pain. A small amount of evidence suggests boswellia may help relieve the inflammation in arthritis, especially when it is combined with an Indian herb called ashwagandha. However, there is little evidence to confirm that it is safe. The recommended dosage is 150mg of boswellia extract, taken three times a day.

Ginger

Ginger root is a traditional remedy for digestive disorders, such as nausea, and arthritic pain. One

GINGER
The root of ginger (*Zingiber officinale*), a plant that is native to southern Asia, is commonly used as a tangy spice. Ground or grated, it can be drunk as a tea or eaten in a variety of sauces, stir-fries, and cakes.

trial showed that ginger eased the pain of osteoarthritis. It may help to relieve pain and inflammation because it seems to block the action of chemicals in the body, such as leukotrienes, that cause pain and swelling.

Cook with ginger regularly but avoid it if you are taking blood thinning drugs, such as warfarin, or if you have gallstones, diabetes, or heart problems – unless your doctor approves.

Bromelain

This protein-digesting enzyme is extracted from the pineapple plant (*Ananas comosus*). Several trials suggest it is an anti-inflammatory and may offer help with pain relief in arthritis. The recommended dosage is 400–600mg of bromelain extract, taken in capsules three

times a day. You should avoid it during pregnancy or while breastfeeding. It may interfere with blood-thinning drugs such as warfarin and large doses may cause stomach upsets.

Turmeric

A spice traditionally used in cookery, turmeric (*Curcuma longa*) has been used in traditional Chinese and Ayurvedic medicine to ease inflammation and pain in arthritis. Small studies suggest that it has an effect when used in combination with other supplements, but there is no scientific evidence that it works alone. High doses of turmeric may act as a blood-thinner and may also cause gastrointestinal upsets. You should avoid turmeric if you have gallstones.

GREEN TEA
Regular consumption of green tea may protect against certain cancers, dental decay, heart disease, kidney stones, and bacterial infections.

Valerian

A couple of scientific trials suggest that valerian may help to promote sleep and relieve anxiety, and so may be useful for those with chronic or acute pain. Do not take valerian with sedatives or hypnotic drugs. Excess valerian may cause serious side-effects.

St John's wort

There is good evidence to suggest that a supplement made from the leaves and stem of St John's wort (*Hypericum perforatum*) can ease the symptoms of mild to moderate depression. However, there is no evidence that it eases the symptoms of arthritis, such as inflammation. Check with your doctor before taking St John's wort as it may interfere with certain medicines and may cause side-effects, such as sensitivity to sunlight, insomnia, and gastrointestinal problems.

Green tea

Drinking green tea may contribute to your general health because of the antioxidants it contains. As yet, there is no firm or conclusive evidence that green tea directly helps to relieve the symptoms of arthritis, although research studies on animals are showing promise.

Burdock

The root of burdock (*Arctium lappa*) helps to remove waste material from inflamed joints and has been used for many conditions, including arthritis. However, there is no convincing scientific evidence that it is effective.

If you suffer from diabetes, always check with your doctor before taking it. Burdock may also affect birth control pills, hormone replacement therapy (HRT), and blood-thinning drugs such as warfarin or heparin.

Trace minerals

You should be able to receive all the trace minerals you need from a balanced diet. However, people with arthritis may benefit from taking extra mineral supplements.

Copper

People who take copper as a supplement or wear it against their skin as a bracelet believe it can relieve pain and inflammation. However, there is no convincing evidence to confirm that this is true. A daily multivitamin supplement will supply you with all the copper you need.

Taking too much copper in supplement form may lead to an overdose, which can be very dangerous, perhaps fatal. Do not wear a magnetic copper bracelet if you are pregnant, have a medical device such as a pacemaker, or are using medication patches.

Selenium

Selenium is a trace mineral that is essential in small amounts for your health. It is found in plants, meat, and seafoods and may be helpful in a number of serious diseases, including cancer, heart disease, and arthritis. Some studies have demonstrated that people with rheumatoid arthritis have lower levels of selenium.

The recommended dose is 50–200 micrograms of selenium, but you should be able to get all you need from a multivitamin supplement. Too much selenium can be toxic.

Manganese

Manganese is a trace mineral that is essential for health. It is found in leafy vegetables, nuts, teas, and wholegrains. There is no evidence that manganese supplements have any effect on arthritis but it may help to keep bones healthy.

Manganese may also affect the absorption of certain drugs, such as antacids, laxatives, and tetracyclines. People with liver failure should avoid it.

Homeopathic medicines

A registered homeopath who is experienced in treating arthritis may recommend one of several medicines to relieve symptoms. Some evidence suggests that these medicines may be effective.

Rhus toxicodendron

Rhus toxicodendron is made from poison ivy and may help with the morning stiffness that affects people with osteoarthritis. If, when you sit for half an hour, your joints rapidly become stiff Rhus toxicodendron may help.

Apis mellifica

Apis mellifica is made from honeybees and may help the hot, swollen, and tender joints that are common in rheumatoid arthritis.

Causticum

Causticum comes from a potassium compound and may help people who have joints that seem to be very sensitive to the weather.

Bodywork therapies

The healing power of touch has been an important part of healthcare since antiquity. Manipulation and bodywork practices, such as massage, chiropractic, and osteopathy, are among the more respected and trustworthy of the complementary therapies. In experienced hands, they aim to ease restrictions, alleviate pain and restore loss of function. At their heart, they are holistic practices that seek to re-balance the body's equilibrium and re-establish the integrated nature of the musculoskeletal system.

Osteopathy, like chiropractic, focuses on the spine and joints, and hinges on the belief that the body has the ability to heal itself.

Chiropractic

Chiropractic is a therapy that focuses on the relationship between the structure of the body, mainly the spine, and overall wellbeing. Aspects of chiropractic have existed for thousands of years, but the modern profession was founded in 1895 by Daniel David Palmer, a Canadian who believed that the body has its own natural healing ability that is controlled by the nervous system.

The spine and other joints, such as the sacro-iliac joints that link the spine to the pelvis, may go out of alignment. Misalignments, or subluxations, of the spine disrupt the nervous system and lead to various complaints and diseases.

Chiropractic has different branches, such as McTimoney chiropractic, but they all continue to highlight the fundamental link between the nervous system and overall health. Chiropractors need a special licence to practise in the UK and undergo training for at least 4 years.

Chiropractors believe the therapy can help with a wide range of conditions, from migraines and back pain to irritable bowel syndrome and asthma. Some evidence suggests that chiropractic can ease acute or chronic lower back pain, but there is no strong evidence that it helps arthritis.

■ **WHAT TO EXPECT AT A CHIROPRACTIC SESSION** Chiropractors will usually begin by discussing your overall health and medical history. They may take X-rays of your spine and will physically examine you, probably in just your underwear, as you sit or lie down.

Chiropractors use a range of different manipulation techniques known as adjustments. Some of these are sharp, jerky movements (known as "high-velocity thrusts") on different parts of the body. You will sometimes hear popping or cracking noises, which are simply the release of tiny air bubbles in the fluid at the surface of a joint. Usually, you will require more than one treatment.

■ **SAFETY ISSUES** Manipulation of inflamed joints and over-exposure to X-rays should be avoided. Consult your GP first if you have osteoporosis, bleeding problems, or a malignant or inflammatory spinal disease.

Osteopathy

Osteopathy, like chiropractic, focuses on the spine and joints, and hinges on the belief that the body has the ability to heal itself. It was pioneered by American doctor Andrew Taylor Still in 1874. Osteopaths work on the premise that misalignments of the skeleton can affect the fluids of the body and lead to a range of conditions, including arthritis.

Osteopaths use manipulation techniques, such as high-velocity thrusts, combined with slightly gentler manoeuvres, including soft-tissue massage, to correct misalignments and let the body heal itself. Osteopaths treat children as well as adults.

The therapy was the first non-conventional therapy in the UK to be regulated by law. Osteopaths undergo a similar amount of training to chiropractors. Your GP may be able to refer you to one.

Osteopathy is used for various conditions, including sciatica, sports injuries, and frozen shoulder. The overall emphasis is on improving mobility, so an osteopath may give you advice on exercise and posture. Some scientific evidence indicates that it can help lower back pain.

■ **WHAT TO EXPECT AT AN OSTEOPATHY SESSION** The osteopath will start by taking your full medical history at the outset. You will need to remove some of your clothes to allow the osteopath to assess the biomechanics of your body, including posture, and to look for excessive strains or weaknesses. Osteopaths rarely use X-rays. The number of sessions you need will depend on your problem.

■ **SAFETY ISSUES** The same as for chiropractic (see above).

SOFT-TISSUE MASSAGE

Massage, in its various forms, can relieve arthritis symptoms such as pain, stiffness, tension, and immobility. The treatment increases blood flow to the muscles to reduce tension, thereby relieving pain and encouraging mobility. However, avoid massage if you are having a flare-up.

THERAPY	WHAT IS IT GOOD FOR?
Swedish massage Involves kneading (petrissage) or rhythmic stroking (effleurage) of muscles and soft tissues; may include oils or electrical stimulation devices.	Reduces general stiffness and releases tension. Benefits osteoarthritis, rheumatoid arthritis, and fibromyalgia.
Chair massage Manipulation in a specially designed chair that bends your body to improve the practitioner's access to your tense joints.	Neck and back joint pain, fibromyalgia, and arthritis pain – so long as you can sit comfortably in the chair.
Myofascial release Slow, gentle manipulation of your fascia – the thin tissues surrounding muscles – to stretch your tense tissues and relieve pain and stress.	Fibromyalgia and general stress relief associated with any chronic illness.
Deep tissue massage Releases tension in deeper layers of soft tissue than Swedish massage, with manipulation across the grain of your muscle; it also may break up scar tissue within the soft tissues.	General arthritis. It is especially good for back pain that is associated with arthritis.

Massage

Massage is one of the oldest forms of complementary therapy and dates back at least as far as ancient Egyptian times. Modern massage, sometimes also known as Swedish massage, was developed in the 19th century by a Swede called Per Henrik Ling. Now there are many different kinds, including massage techniques that are gentler than Ling's quite vigorous methods. There are various soft-tissue massage techniques (see Soft-tissue Massage, left), some of which may also use aromatherapy oils (see p.124).

Massage is used for a wide range of conditions – from back pain and fibromylagia to irritable bowel syndrome, headaches, and general stress relief – and the evidence to support its use is relatively good.

■ **WHAT TO EXPECT AT A MASSAGE SESSION** You will usually have to take off some clothes before the massage starts. The therapist will use a variety of rubbing, stroking, pressing, or kneading techniques that may be vigorous and stimulating, or gentle and relaxing, or a combination of both. During the massage, the therapist may use creams, oils, or talcum powder.

■ **SAFETY ISSUES** Avoid massage if you have a flare-up. Anyone with deep vein thrombosis, burns, skin diseases or infections, open wounds, osteoporosis, or bone fractures should seek medical advice before receiving a massage.

Rolfing

Rolfing is a deep pressure form of massage that was developed in the 1950s by Dr Ida Rolf, who believed that releasing muscle tension would lead to overall health. Rolfing is also referred to as "structural integration" and is used for general stress relief, headaches, and back pain. However, there is no strong evidence that it works.

■ **WHAT TO EXPECT AT A ROLFING SESSION** There will be similarities with other forms of massage, but the techniques are often more forceful and probing.

■ **SAFETY ISSUES** Damage may be caused to those with rheumatoid arthritis or other inflammatory joint disorders. Avoid any painful or uncomfortable massage if you have a flare-up in your condition. (See also Massage, opposite.)

Reiki

Reiki is a touch therapy that originated in Japan at the start of the 20th century. It is based on the idea that good health comes from a balanced "energy flow" in the body. Reiki in Japanese translates as "universal energy" and the therapist aims to use this universal energy to improve your personal energy flow. Reiki is used as a general therapy to ease stress or promote relaxation, but there is no scientific evidence that it works.

■ **WHAT TO EXPECT AT A REIKI SESSION** You sit or lie down but do not usually need to remove any clothes. The therapist then lays both hands gently on different parts of your body.

■ **SAFETY ISSUES** There are no known safety issues.

Acupuncture

Acupuncture is perhaps the most ancient of all the complementary therapies; Chinese texts refer to it from the first century BC, but it is probably older still.

Acupuncture is based on the belief that good health comes from a perfect balance between two opposites – *yin* and *yang*. Diseases or health complaints occur because of an imbalance between *yin* and *yang*, which upsets the flow of the body's vital energy, known as *qi* (pronounced "chee"). This energy moves through the body along meridians, which form a network of 12 pathways that feature more than 350 acupoints.

Acupuncturists insert tiny needles into specific acupoints to adjust the flow of *qi* and rebalance the *yin* and *yang*. Practitioners of acupressure, or a similar therapy called shiatsu, use their fingers and hands instead of needles.

ACUPUNCTURE TREATMENT
An acupuncturist inserts a needle into the tissue just below the skin. The treatment may require the acupuncturist to insert needles into several acupoints.

Acupuncture is not legally restricted and many mainstream surgeries and pain clinics offer it with conventional treatments.

Acupuncture can be used for many conditions, including pain from osteoarthritis, fibromylagia, nausea, headache, depression, and back pain. However, the evidence for its effectiveness is mixed and depends on the condition: there is strong evidence for dental pain and nausea, promising evidence for fibromyalgia, but conflicting evidence for treating back pain and osteoarthritis. Nevertheless, acupuncture has been shown to cause the brain to release certain chemicals called endorphins that may ease pain.

■ **WHAT TO EXPECT AT AN ACUPUNCTURE SESSION** In the first session, the acupuncturist will discuss your health complaint and take your full medical history before deciding on treatment.

The acupuncturist inserts a series of long, thin, disposable needles just under the surface of the skin at various acupoints that may be on the face and scalp. This does not usually hurt, although some people may experience a little discomfort, such as a tingling sensation at the site of the needles. The needles are left in for a few seconds or up to 20 minutes.

■ **SAFETY ISSUES** People with a severe bleeding disorder should not receive acupuncture.

ESSENTIAL OILS

Aromatherapy oils, also known as essential oils, are often used in massage. They come from plant essences, have unique properties, and may be applied directly to the skin in a carrier oil, inhaled with steam, or used to scent a room via a diffuser. The evidence of their efficacy is inconclusive, although some oils have been found to help anxiety, relieve insomnia, or combat fungi.

OIL	WHAT IS IT GOOD FOR?
Lavender	General relaxation. Aid for insomnia, stress, or anxiety.
Marjoram, Spanish	To promote relaxation and ease muscle fatigue.
Rosemary	To reduce pain and swelling and improve circulation.
Thyme	To ease joint pain.
Ylang ylang	For anxiety and insomnia.
Chamomile	To ease muscle and rheumatic pain and promote relaxation.

Aromatherapy

Aromatherapy is renowned for its ability to help increase vitality, improve wellbeing, and restore health. Its unique oils can help with various ailments (see left).

The basic principles are straightforward, which makes aromatherapy a good candidate for self-treatment at home. You can massage the oils into your skin, inhale them, or add them to a bath. However, you will get the best treatment from a professional aromatherapist.

■ **WHAT TO EXPECT AT AN AROMATHERAPY SESSION** You will be asked about your past and present state of health, and also about your diet and lifestyle. The therapist will select suitable oils, ask you to remove some of your clothes, and then give you a massage using the oils.

■ **SAFETY ISSUES** Check with your GP before using any essential oils in the first three months of pregnancy. Always check with your GP before using oils on children. Large quantities of any oil may be dangerous and they should never be directly ingested.

Reflexology

Reflexology is a therapy that focuses on the feet and sometimes the hands. The modern form of reflexology was developed in the early 20th century by William Fitzgerald, an American ear, nose, and throat specialist.

The idea is that zones on the soles of the feet, or palms of the hands, reflect corresponding organs and parts of the body. By massaging the zones in a selective way, a reflexologist can remove blockages of energy and so ease or even cure various ailments.

Reflexology may benefit many disorders, but is most often used for stress relief, arthritis, irritable bowel syndrome, headaches, and premenstrual problems. The evidence for its effectiveness is not conclusive though some evidence suggests it can help headaches and premenstrual problems.

■ **WHAT TO EXPECT AT A REFLEXOLOGY SESSION** After giving your detailed medical history, you will need to take off your shoes and socks and may either sit or lie down. By applying finger and thumb pressure, the reflexologist will massage selected areas of your feet, and occasionally your hands.

Treatment does not usually feel ticklish – in fact, most people find it very relaxing, although some of the strokes can be quite firm and intense. You can expect to have several sessions, usually one a week for 6 weeks.

■ **SAFETY ISSUES** People with bone or joint problems in the feet should be treated with extra care.

REFLEXOLOGY MASSAGE
A reflexologist uses thumb or finger pressure to massage particular areas of the feet.

Movement therapies

Keeping mobile is very important for people with arthritis (see p.158). When your joints are stiff or sore, it is often tempting to avoid using them, but this can lead to greater pain and disability. Movement therapies, such as yoga, tai chi, and the Alexander technique, are about learning new ways of holding, stretching, and moving your body. These changes will bring about improvements to your posture that might not only ease symptoms, but lead to an overall sensation of wellbeing.

Osteopaths and chiropractors often recommend Pilates to people who suffer from back problems because it focuses on core strength, which means toning and strengthening the abdomen.

Yoga

The practice of yoga focuses on unifying the mind, body, and spirit in a way that is claimed to bring good health and a relaxed state of mind. There are many different types of yoga, ranging from the relaxing to the very challenging.

In the West, the most commonly practised type of yoga is hatha yoga, which is based around poses (asanas), meditation, and breath control (pranayama). Yoga teachers will show you how to stretch and hold your body in the different poses and how to practise breathing and meditation.

■ **WHO IS YOGA SUITABLE FOR?** Yoga may be suitable for everyone and whether or not you have arthritis. Check with your doctor first and if yoga suits you, be prepared to practise it regularly.

■ **HOW MIGHT YOGA HELP ME?** Yoga has been shown to improve mood and wellbeing. Specifically, it may help those with high blood pressure and joint stiffness. One study found that it eased the symptoms of rheumatoid arthritis.

■ **SAFETY ISSUES** Choose the right level for your needs and don't over-extend yourself. Try to find a qualified instructor who can teach yoga to people with arthritis.

Pilates

This technique focuses on a series of exercises designed to strengthen the body, improve flexibility and help with overall posture. It also involves concentration and learning to breathe in a controlled, supposedly beneficial way. The exercises may be carried out on mats at home or in a class, or by using special apparatus in a Pilates studio. There are several different forms, each based on the exercises developed by Joseph Pilates in the early 1920s in Germany.

■ **WHO IS PILATES SUITABLE FOR?** Pilates is suitable for anyone, including the elderly, pregnant women, and people with arthritis. It is important to choose the right level for your needs.

■ **HOW MIGHT PILATES HELP ME?**
Osteopaths and chiropractors often recommend Pilates to people who suffer from back problems because it focuses on core strength, which means toning and strengthening the abdomen.

Pilates can also help you correctly align your pelvis and spine. The movements are quite gentle and slow although they can become much more difficult as you progress and develop strength. One study shows that it may help joint mobility, but there is no research into its effects on arthritis.

■ **SAFETY ISSUES** Pilates is relatively gentle and should not present any safety concerns. As with all forms of exercise, avoid movements that feel painful, particularly if you have inflamed joints.

PRACTICAL TIPS

SAFETY ISSUES

In all movement therapies, make sure you:

● Choose the right level and don't over-extend yourself.

● Only move your body and limbs within a range that is comfortable for you – your comfort zone. There is no place for the notion of "no pain, no gain".

● Stop at once if any movement feels painful or uncomfortable.

● Tell your instructor, before you begin a class, that you have arthritis and explain how you are affected by it.

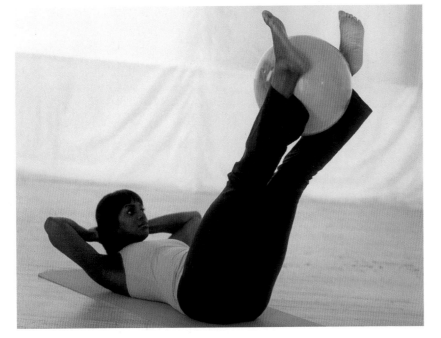

PRACTISING PILATES
Special equipment is not essential for practising Pilates at home, although a mat, a rolled-up towel, and a sizeable ball are useful.

Tai chi

Tai chi is a system of movements and postures with roots in both martial arts and ancient Chinese philosophy. It is designed to improve strength and flexibility, and promote wellbeing through bodily harmony. Like acupuncture (see p.123), tai chi embodies the principle that disharmony between the forces of *yin* and *yang* lead to health complaints, including pain and disease.

Tai chi is taught in small classes in which certain slow movements are combined with deep breathing and concentration. If tai chi suits you, be prepared to practise it for a short while each day and to make it a lifelong commitment.

■ **WHO IS TAI CHI SUITABLE FOR?** Tai chi is suitable for everyone, including elderly people and people with arthritis.

■ **HOW MIGHT TAI CHI HELP ME?** Tai chi is an easy technique to learn, can relieve pain and stress, and brings inner peace. It helps to align your spine and takes many of your joints through their normal range of movement.

Tai chi has been shown to help with developing balance and strength in a way that improves confidence and reduces falls in elderly people. It has also helped

TAI CHI OUTDOORS
Each day, Chinese people gather outdoors, in the park or in the street, to practise the sequences of tai chi.

people with depression and fatigue and can improve the function of the heart and lungs of elderly people. A trial of elderly women with osteoarthritis of the knee also showed that they benefited from learning tai chi.

■ **SAFETY ISSUES** Consult your doctor before you start and speak to the instructor first.

Qi gong

Qi gong is a traditional Chinese technique that combines meditation and movement to build stamina and ease the stress of chronic conditions.

■ **WHO IS QI GONG SUITABLE FOR?** Like tai chi, Qi gong is suitable for everyone, including elderly people and people with arthritis.

■ **HOW MIGHT QI GONG HELP ME?** Qi gong is used in traditional Chinese medicine for many

Tai chi is taught in small classes in which certain slow movements are combined with deep breathing and concentration.

Q&A

Will the movements of tai chi help me to fight my arthritis?

Try not to think in terms of "fighting" your disease – you are not being "attacked", nor do you have to "conquer" your condition. Although tai chi has its roots in martial arts, its movements are graceful, not aggressive. They will encourage you to focus your physical and mental energies in a way that helps you protect your health.

medical conditions. Some evidence suggests that Qi gong may help people with high blood pressure, although the research is limited.

Qi gong may help you relax, which could in theory help with the management of pain or stress, but there is no hard scientific evidence to support this.

■ **SAFETY ISSUES** Try to find a qualified instructor who can teach Qi gong to people with arthritis. Rarely, the symptoms of people with psychiatric conditions may get worse. If you have a psychiatric disorder, speak to your doctor before trying Qi gong.

CORRECTING BAD POSTURE
A practitioner of the Alexander technique can help you to undo your postural bad habits and to learn new ways of sitting and standing that avoid tension.

Alexander technique

The Alexander technique is a way of learning to correctly hold and move your body so that you can improve your posture, balance, and co-ordination. Australian actor Frederick Alexander developed the technique at the start of the 20th century after he suffered problems with his voice.

After observing himself in a mirror, he realized that he was holding his neck in a tense position and wondered if this was the root of his trouble. He gradually worked on solving the problem by devising a series of movements that altered the way he held his head, neck, and spine.

The Alexander technique is often taught in drama schools as a way of helping students learn to move and use their bodies freely, and to help with voice problems. The technique is also used by some sports people.

■ **HOW MIGHT THE ALEXANDER TECHNIQUE HELP ME?** The technique is based on the idea that the head, neck, and spine play a crucial role in the overall flexibility and health of the body. Over the years, you have probably developed awkward ways of sitting, standing, and moving. You unconsciously tense up with anxiety or stress and adopt poor postures that affect the way you move your body.

Alexander teachers work with people on a one-to-one basis and gently use their hands to show you how to correct postural problems and to learn to use your body in the most "natural" way.

The technique has been shown to benefit people with respiratory problems and back pain, and to work on the body's autonomic nervous system to help relieve stress and anxiety.

■ **SAFETY ISSUES** Consult your doctor before you start.

Feldenkrais method

This therapy is like the Alexander technique in that it teaches you patterns of movement that help to ease your health complaints and maximize your flexibility. The method was developed by Israeli physicist Moshe Feldenkrais after he suffered a serious knee injury.

In a small class, known as Awareness Through Movement, you learn to practise a series of gentle movements that you can do while sitting, standing, or lying down. Alternatively, you can have one-to-one consultations, known as Functional Integration, in which the teacher uses his or her hands to guide you directly. You may also receive a massage.

■ **HOW MIGHT THE FELDENKRAIS METHOD HELP ME?** People may learn the Feldenkrais method for many reasons, such as rehabilitation after an accident, alleviating anxiety and stress, or relieving pain. There is

evidence that it may have mild benefits for low back pain, and also for shoulder and neck pain.

■ **SAFETY ISSUES** There are no known safety issues, but if you have suffered an injury or are recovering from surgery, consult your doctor first.

Trager approach

Proponents of the Trager approach believe that ill-health and stress stem from the unconscious mind. The method was developed in America by Milton Trager, a boxer turned doctor who realized that a range of movements and touch techniques can change unhealthy mental and physical habits.

A session of Trager work will involve you lying on a padded table in a semi-meditative state while the therapist moves your body in certain ways, using rocking, gentle shaking, or stretching techniques.

You can also practise a series of mental exercises, known as "Mentastics", at home. One example involves you shifting the way you hold your weight in order to maintain a "freer" body.

■ **HOW MIGHT THE TRAGER APPROACH HELP ME?** Very little research exists, although one study has shown that the Trager approach may benefit people with back pain.

■ **SAFETY ISSUES** Consult your doctor before you start.

Alexander teachers work with people on a one-to-one basis and gently use their hands to show you how to correct postural problems and to learn to use your body in the most "natural" way.

Living with arthritis

If you have been diagnosed with arthritis you will need to make changes to the way you live your life. How extensive those changes become will depend on the type of arthritis you have and how it is affecting you. People with a mild condition may only need to make minor adjustments, while those who are affected more severely may find that there are many challenges to address.

Occupational therapists, physiotherapists, and many other specialists can provide you with a great deal of advice and guidance to help you manage your arthritis and deal with issues that arise in everyday life. Such issues include the impact of arthritis on your work, domestic activities, driving, family life, and personal relationships.

One aspect of arthritis that can be hard is not knowing how long it is going to last or when it is going to flare up into an episode of pain, inflammation, and swelling. Coping with these episodes can be stressful, so it is good to learn and practise techniques that not only help you get through the pain and stress, but also protect your joints from potential damage.

Day-to-day living

The pain, stiffness, and other symptoms of your arthritis can have a profound impact on the way you go about your day-to-day living. Your work may be compromised and your domestic life may become a daily challenge. But there is no reason to despair because there is usually help at hand. Laws protect your rights at work, occupational therapists can help you solve your practical problems, and friends and family will give you plenty of support. For those who cherish their independence, a whole host of clever assistive devices and energy-saving tips are available to make your life much easier.

It is important to identify and sort out potential problems as early as possible.

Working

If you are diagnosed with arthritis, one of your first concerns may be how your job or your chances of getting one are affected. Questions may surround your finances, how sympathetic your employer will be, or how you are going to perform some aspects of your job.

First of all, don't panic. Various people and organizations can help if you are having difficulties (see Who Can Help?, p.135). In the UK, legislation also gives you certain rights. If, for example, you have rheumatoid arthritis, don't worry about being sacked because

of your condition. The Disability Discrimination Act (1995) states that your employer is responsible for making reasonable accommodations to your current job or considering you for suitable vacancies within the company. You also have some responsibilities under the Health and Safety Act (1974), such as taking reasonable care for your own and others' health and safety at work.

Modifying the workplace
If arthritis does not compromise your job excessively, it is important to identify and sort out potential problems as early as possible.

If you can't, seek independent advice (see Who Can Help?, right).

Under the law, your place of employment should be accessible to anyone with a disability. Your employer also has a duty to make "reasonable accommodations" that will not cause disproportionate disruption and that are affordable. Examples of these include:

• Changes to your working environment, such as ergonomic changes to your work station, doors that open automatically, an allocated parking space, and suitable building alterations.

• Changes to your duties.

• Change to your timetable, such as new working hours, flexible working, and change of shifts.

• The purchase of modified equipment and assistive devices, such as a chunky pen, a dictaphone, or voice-activated software if writing is difficult.

• The assignment of a support worker to work with you to get the job done.

Returning to work

If you have been off work – for surgery or a flare-up, for example – a successful return can depend on a number of factors, including the nature of your job, the severity of your arthritis, and how long you have been away.

Tell your employer about your arthritis and discuss the kind of changes you will need. Suggest a graded return in terms of a build-up of hours and responsibilities and ask for a regular review. If you can only manage fewer hours, estimate the minimum you need to live on. Your occupational therapist can give support and the Disability Employment Advisor can give you advice (see Who Can Help?, below).

WHO CAN HELP?

You and your manager may be able to solve the workplace problems yourselves. If you need extra help, the following people and organizations can give you advice, information and/or practical help about working with arthritis. You need to get as much information and advice as possible to help you cope and if necessary to make an informed decision about your future.

PROFESSIONAL	WHAT'S ON OFFER
Occupational health provider	Ask to be referred for an occupational health assessment. Most companies and organizations have doctors and some nurses; a few also employ counsellors, physiotherapists, and occupational therapists, so it is worth asking for an appointment with one of them.
Healthcare professional (GP, rheumatologist, etc.)	Advice and information.
Rheumatology occupational therapist	Advice and information on work issues. Some may offer an enhanced service, such as carrying out a work assessment, work report with recommendations, meeting with your employer, etc.
Disability Employment Advisor (DEA)	Works at your local Jobcentre and gives advice and support. Ask for a work assessment. Can put you in touch with other government work schemes.
Access to Work advisor	Scheme operated through Jobcentre Plus that gives practical and financial support, including funding for equipment, alteration to work environment, help with transport costs, or a provision of a support worker. Ask the DEA for more information.

Household chores

The bending, lifting, pushing, gripping, and carrying involved in doing household chores can take their toll on sore and aching joints and leave you with little energy to spare for your more enjoyable leisure activities.

Think of easier ways of doing things. Try sitting while you are preparing food. Use energy-saving equipment, such as a microwave or electric tin opener.

Well-designed tools require less effort to use and are less stressful for your joints. A good example is the chunky grip on hand tools, such as a chopping knife and a screwdriver, or on lever door handles and taps. If you have painful wrists or knees, wear a supportive splint.

■ **CLEANING** Try keeping an upright posture, bending your knees rather than your back, and don't try to clean the whole house in one go! A lightweight, upright vacuum cleaner may be easier to use. Check you can grip the handle, operate the controls, and change the bags easily before you buy one. Ask someone to carry the vacuum cleaner upstairs for you or, better still, keep another one up there permanently.

Bending to pick items off the floor can be difficult. A pick-up stick or long-handled dustpan and brush can be useful. To save on trips upstairs when tidying up, collect items in a basket at the bottom of the stairs and take them up in one go.

■ **LAUNDRY** Front-loading washing machines and tumble driers are easier to reach if mounted on a firm plinth. If you prefer pegging out clothes on a line to dry, use push-on dolly pegs rather than squeeze-open pegs. If you find reaching up difficult, try propping up your clothes line with a forked

COPING WITH HOUSEWORK

Cleaning, tidying, making meals, doing the laundry, ironing, and all those other chores that constitute household work can be tiring at the best of times. There are a number of tips that will conserve your energy, protect your joints, and generally make your life a good deal easier.

TIP	ACTIVITY
Plan ahead	Make a list of household jobs and plan to do a little over several days, rather than all at once. Plan rest days and make a list of potential helpers.
Pace yourself	Take regular breaks when doing housework. Be systematic and avoid unnecessary trips around the house and upstairs.
Posture and position	Keep a relaxed upright posture, bending from the knees rather than the back. Change position often and avoid gripping things tightly for long periods – for example, when polishing or scrubbing pans.
Get help	Ask family or friends to help with heavier tasks. You may be able to pay for someone to do the cleaning for you.
Storage	Store items that you often use at the front of cupboards at chest height. Throw away old bottles you no longer use and keep cupboards uncluttered.

stick. The line can be let down
to peg on the clothes and then
raised up to dry.

When ironing, wear a wrist
support, use a lightweight iron,
and sit on a stool (see p.176).
Iron a little at a time and if you
have room, leave the board
standing. Many man-made fabrics
do not need to be ironed at all.

■ **MAKING BEDS** Stretchy man-made
fabrics, fitted sheets, and
lightweight duvets may be easier
to manage. Velcro fastenings on
covers are kinder to hands than
press studs.

■ **MEAL PREPARATION** If you cook
often, and you can afford them,
buy lightweight power tools to
stir, chop, grate, and whisk food.
Use a knife and vegetable peeler
with a chunky grip.

Choose appliances, such as a
cooker and a microwave, that you
can reach into and that feature
easy-to-operate controls. Use
lightweight pans for cooking,
preferably with two handles.

To avoid lifting pans of boiling
water, steam or microwave your
vegetables. If you use a saucepan,
put a chip basket in the pan.
When the vegetables are done
you can remove the basket and
leave the pan of water to cool.
Alternatively, use a slotted spoon.

If you do not eat in the kitchen,
a trolley can be helpful to take
food through to another room.
Keep some frozen meals at hand
for "bad days".

■ **WASHING UP** Most items will go in a
dishwasher, but if you wash up
and dry by hand, rest the pans in
the sink or on the draining board.
If you have to stoop over the sink,
reduce the amount you have to
bend by placing an upturned bowl
under your washing-up bowl.

■ **SHOPPING** Internet shopping and
home-delivery services have made
this job easier for many people.
Most supermarkets will pack
groceries and take them to your
car. They also have clip-on trolleys
for wheelchairs. Shop-mobility
and disabled parking schemes
are available in most areas.

■ **IN THE WORKSHOP AND GARDEN** By
adapting the ideas mentioned
above, you can successfully garden
and carry out maintenance tasks.

PICK-UP STICK
You can avoid the pain of bending
down to pick things up off the
floor if you use a pick-up stick.

SOLVING EVERYDAY PROBLEMS

Many assistive devices are either based on common sense or are the result of ingenious solutions. They are all derived from tried-and-tested ways of helping you solve manual problems and accomplish everyday activities that are normal for people who do not have arthritis.

ACTIVITY	PROBLEM	SOLUTION
Writing	Weak grip because of painful wrist and fingers.	Use a pen with a chunky, rubber grip and try to relax your grip on the pen as you write.
Peeling potatoes	Gripping and turning the peeler.	Choose a wide-handled peeler (available in high-street stores).
Washing and drying feet, neck, and back	Reaching becomes difficult due to pain.	Wash with a long-handled sponge. Dry with a lightweight towel that has hand loops. Wear a towelling bathrobe.
Turning a key	Gripping and turning a key.	Fit a handle to your key to give you better leverage.
Picking up things from the floor	Reaching down.	Use a pick-up stick (see p.137).

Splints

Wearing a splint can support and protect unstable and painful joints in your body, such as the wrists, hands, fingers, knees, and ankles. Splints can help you with walking, gripping, handling objects, and in easing the pain and swelling of arthritis. You can either buy them ready made "off the shelf" or you can ask an occupational therapist or a physiotherapist to make a splint specially for you.

Home modifications

You may wish to modify your home in order to improve your ability to get around. For example, if you have arthritis in your hips, knees, or ankles, you may have difficulty rising from a seat or climbing steps and stairs.

If your shoulders or hands are affected, you may find that reaching into cupboards, plugging in electrical appliances, or turning on taps is a problem.

Getting into and around your home

A grab rail beside the front or back door will help you manage the steps into your home. You may need a ramp – a gradient of 1 in 12 is recommended if you are a wheelchair user. For the stairs, an extra banister rail may be all you need to steady yourself. There are many types of stair lift on the market for those who need more help and a through-floor lift will benefit wheelchair users.

If you use a walking frame or wheelchair indoors, you will need a little more space to allow you to turn in a room and to move from one room to another. Removing an internal wall can improve your access and mobility in the home.

Help with rising

People with arthritis find that a chair designed with a high seat and back as well as arm rests is relaxing to sit in. It is also easier to get up from such a chair than from a low three-piece suite. You can raise the seat of your chair by placing a deep cushion on it or by fitting a purpose-made chair raise unit under it. A powered riser-recliner chair with an elevating leg rest is ideal.

Your toilet may be raised by building a plinth under it or by fitting it with a purpose-made, raised toilet seat. These come with or without rails. Alternatively, a grab rail fitted to the wall may help you rise from the toilet. If arthritis affects your arms and hands, toilets can be equipped with a washing and drying facility.

Beds can be raised on blocks to help you stand up when you get up. A rail fitted to the bed can help you sit up from a lying-down position. For even more assistance, try using a powered pillow or mattress lifter.

Taking a shower is easier than getting out of a bath and a walk-in shower is easiest to access. A grab rail on the wall or a seat can be helpful in a shower or a bath. If you prefer to soak in a warm bath and need more help to get out, try a power-rise bath seat, with or without a reclining back rest.

Ergonomic design

A good ergonomic design in the home may involve altering the height of work surfaces and cupboards, raising or lowering appliances and electric sockets

Wearing a splint can support and protect unstable and painful joints in your body.

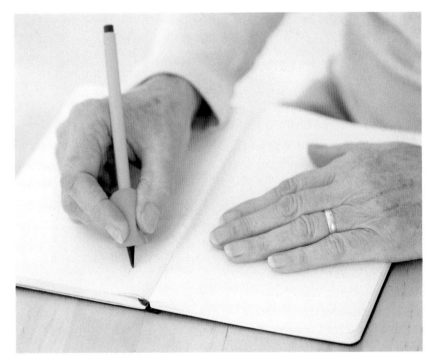

PEN GRIP
Writing becomes easier with a pen grip because you don't have to press hard and you feel less pain and fatigue.

PRACTICAL TIPS

CHOOSING ASSISTIVE DEVICES

- Look for lightweight, well-designed products that have a good grip and easy-to-operate controls.

- Chunky grips or handles increase leverage and help if you have a weak grip.

- Consider the posture you will need to adopt to use it. For example, a vacuum cleaner with an upright handle will be easier on your back than one that requires you to stoop.

- Ask an occupational therapist to help pick what you need and to show you how to use it.

- Ask specialist equipment shops and Disabled Living Centres for advice.

- Try before you buy and shop around if you can. Make sure mail order products are returnable if they are unsuitable.

to enable you to gain access, and ensuring controls and handles are easy to grip. The sink, cooker, and work surface of your kitchen's "working triangle" should be close together, at the same height, and without obstruction.

Assistive devices

Using assistive devices or gadgets will help you to cope with the difficulties arthritis can cause. They may be familiar products that you can find in any high-street shop or specifically designed to help overcome a disability.

For example, electric tin openers are widely available and reduce the effort required by a manual gadget. However, you will need to find a specialist shop or supplier to purchase a sock aid (which helps put socks on when you cannot reach your feet).

The Disabled Living Foundation can advise on equipment and aids. Social services may loan you larger items of specialist equipment.

Personal care

Pain and stiffness in shoulders, back, and hips can make it hard to reach down to put on shoes and socks, or to reach up to brush your hair or put clothes over your head.

Various long-handled gadgets will help with most problems – for example, long-handled shoe horn, sponge, hair brush, and "helping

hand". A stick with a hook at one end and a rubber thimble at the other can help hook pants over your feet or push shirts off your shoulders. It is best to choose clothing with few fastenings if your grip is weak.

A button hook can be helpful and tying a loop on a zip gives a better grip. Choose chunky grips or use an electric toothbrush or razor. Try moist toilet tissue if using ordinary is difficult.

General household needs

A wide range of gadgets is available to help you with many of your general household needs:

- Jar, bottle, and tin openers.
- Wide-handled peelers, chunky cutlery, and ergonomic knives with upright handles.
- Lever gadgets for taps, door handles, keys, and plugs.
- Long-handled dustpan and brush.
- Kettle tippers.
- Self-opening scissors.

LONG-HANDLED DUSTPAN AND BRUSH

Long-handles so you can stand upright.

Dust pan swivels so you don't need to bend over.

MULTI-CHOPPER

Press top
to chop.

FRUIT AND VEGETABLE PEELER

Swivel blade
can be used
right- or left-
handed.

Place herbs
or vegetables
in the base.

Chunky, easy-
grip handle

Clip to keep
closed when
not in use.

SELF-OPENING SCISSORS

Spring to
force open
blades.

Chunky
handle

JAR AND BOTTLE OPENER

Slide over
jar lid.

Teeth grip
lid to make
turning easy.

Chunky, easy-
grip handle

- Contour grips to turn both knobs and dials.
- Book rests and pen grips.
- Wrist rests, adapted keyboards, and mouse control for computers.

Family life and looking after children

Raising a family can be the most rewarding and productive time in life. Families make many physical and emotional demands, however. Pain, fatigue, and disability caused by arthritis can combine to interfere with your role as an active parent.

A survey of grandparents and parents with arthritis revealed that the most common childcare problems were lifting up a baby or child from the floor or from a cot, encouraging children to help with household chores, and having enough energy to keep up with children (see Looking After Babies and Children, right).

Arthritis has an impact on how family members feel about and relate to one another, how roles and responsibilities are taken on, and how decisions are made.

If you are a parent with arthritis, you may feel guilty about being unable to do all the things you think you should for your family. You may not be able to walk your children to school, play football with them because your knees are painful, or go out with your partner because you feel too tired.

At the same time, the pain and inflammation you feel may make you more irritable and you may take it out on those nearest you, or push them away when they offer help or comfort.

Family members who are usually eager to help you can unwittingly contribute to your feelings of helplessness, frustration, and dependence. This is especially true when they jump in too quickly and immediately take

KITCHEN TOOLS
A range of kitchen tools makes many food preparation tasks easier and less painful.

PRACTICAL TIPS

LOOKING AFTER BABIES AND CHILDREN

- Make sure you can use baby equipment safely and manage the fastenings.

- Change nappies where you don't need to stoop.

- When bathing a baby use a sculpted foam cushion and nonslip mat. On "bad" days, just use a mat and a sponge.

- Manage your energy so you have enough for play.

- Get children to help you by making household tasks into a game.

- Read books together – it allows you to rest.

- Encourage children to climb gently onto your knee.

PRACTICAL TIPS

SEXUAL RELATIONSHIPS

● Paying attention to your whole being is important in being attractive to others.

● Make time for yourself and your lover.

● Pamper yourself – go to the hairdressers, get a manicure, meet up for a meal, go away together.

● Take your medication before sexual activity to be as pain-free as possible.

● Take a hot shower or bath before sexual activity to relax joints and muscles.

● Consider the most convenient method of contraception for you both.

● Discover together the most appropriate sexual positions. You may need to develop other ways to please each other when intercourse is not possible.

● Ask a health professional or a sexual counsellor you trust if you cannot resolve your problems.

● Remember – it's good to talk so keep the lines of communication open!

over all the jobs that you are finding difficult or painful. You will need to negotiate the amount of help you want so that you can keep some of your independence.

Your family can be a major source of emotional and practical support and it is very important to communicate honestly with them. Just as you may have had difficulty accepting that you have arthritis, your family may find it difficult to come to terms with, too. Explain to them about arthritis and how you feel, and encourage them to ask questions. This will help them to see past the problems to the real you and help them come to terms with their loss.

Personal relationships

Arthritis does not just affect you in isolation – it can potentially affect everyone who comes into contact with you. Good communication is the key to maintaining all your relationships, whether platonic or sexual. For people with arthritis this is equally, if not more, vital.

Communication takes effort and when you are in pain or feeling tired you may find you don't have the energy. Be honest about how you feel – those closest to you need to know. Sometimes it is hard to explain your arthritis, so give an information leaflet to your family and work colleagues.

A LOVING RELATIONSHIP
People with arthritis can expect to share in the joy and pleasure of a loving relationship.

The differences between the types of arthritis are not understood very well. Ask your doctor or Arthritis Care (see Useful Addresses, p.215) for a leaflet.

Sexuality and sexual relationships

Sexuality is an important part of who we are. We express this in different ways: in the way we dress, present ourselves, and communicate – both verbally and non-verbally. Many people express themselves within a sexual relationship. Arthritis can have a negative impact on your sexuality and sexual relationships and so it is important that you address issues as they arise (see Sexual Relationships, p.142).

Travelling and moving around

Pain and fatigue can restrict your independence and reduce the frequency and length of time you can spend travelling. The following advice can help you improve your ability to get around:

■ **COMFORTABLE FOOTWEAR** Make sure your footwear gives you the maximum amount of comfort. Trainers or thick-soled shoes are best. It can be difficult to find footwear that looks good and is comfortable. Ask your podiatrist (chiropodist), health professional, or a good shoe shop for advice.

■ **WALKING AIDS** Various types of walking aids are available. There are special handles that can reduce the stress on hand and upper limb joints that are affected by arthritis. It is best to get advice from a physiotherapist, who will be able to tell you what walking aids are most suitable for you.

■ **WHEELCHAIRS AND SCOOTERS** The perception that wheelchairs and scooters are often considered a last resort is understandable. They can, however, provide you with valuable independence and increase your opportunities to travel and socialize.

Standard manual or electric wheelchairs can be provided by the NHS but if you want non-standard models then you may need to buy them privately. You can make an appointment at your local Disabled Living Centre if you need advice and an opportunity to try various products before you buy from a manufacturer.

■ **DRIVING** Driving can be a real challenge, depending on the type of car you have, how far you are travelling, and the severity of your arthritis. Ask your doctor to refer you to your nearest Driving Assessment Centre.

Speak to your health or social service professional or contact the Department of Work and Pensions because you may be eligible for a Motability car through the Disability Living Allowance if you are receiving a high-rate mobility

WALKING AIDS
Various sturdy walking aids can help to provide support, stability, and balance.

Your family can be a major source of emotional and practical support.

component. Contact your local Customs and Excise office because you may also be eligible for help with road tax costs.

If travelling by car is difficult, some tips can make the journey easier. For instance, it may help to take your painkillers and/or anti-inflammatory drugs at a particular time before you start so they are working effectively when you most need them. Try a wrist support whilst driving if you have problems with your wrist or grip. Take plenty of breaks during the journey.

■ **TRAINS, BOATS AND PLANES** These forms of transport can be more relaxing and less stressful than driving a car, especially on long journeys. Train stations, ferry terminals, and airports should be accessible under the Disability Discrimination Act 1995 for people with a disability. It is always worth ringing ahead to your travel provider to say what assistance you are likely to need.

Occupational therapists

People with arthritis can turn to an occupational therapist for help in achieving their personal, work, domestic, educational, or leisure goals. Occupational therapists can help you improve your ability to carry out routine tasks, make lifestyle changes, and prevent or reduce your chances of losing roles and abilities in the future.

Q&A

I have great difficulty parking my car near to the shops – what help can I get?

The European Blue Badge permits special parking allowances to people with disabilities. In the UK, these badges are normally issued automatically if you are claiming the high-rate mobility component of the Disability Living Allowance.

A rheumatologist can refer you to a rheumatology occupational therapist who specializes in solving the problems of arthritis. Either on your own or through a referral from your health professional, you can contact the occupational therapists at the local social services for advice on larger equipment or home adaptations.

How occupational therapists can help

Occupational therapists can help in a number of ways, usually when you are in hospital or when you are at home. Some may see you at a school or university, or at work. Occupational therapists can advise you on everything covered in this chapter – from household chores, home modifications, and assistive devices, to work, travel, asking for help, family life, and childcare.

Usually, occupational therapists will assess and treat you on a one-to-one basis. However, they may prefer to invite you to attend group sessions. Occupational therapists can help you by:

- Discussing practical problems and showing you how you can overcome them. These could include problems at home, work, school, and further education or with your leisure pursuits.
- Teaching you how to look after your joints. It is important that you understand as much as possible how arthritis affects your joints and what you can do in your day-to-day activities to get the most out of them. This includes teaching you how to minimize the strain you put on your joints.
- Teaching you physical or psychological techniques to manage your pain and fatigue.
- Helping you to return to former activities or teaching new activities to help you achieve your goals.
- Making splints to rest or support painful or damaged joints.

Asking for help

Ask for what you need – it will improve your chances of getting it. When you have arthritis, you don't have to battle alone. Acknowledge your limitations and accept help without feeling guilty. Having someone do the jobs that hurt or make you tired will save you energy and reduce frustration. Friends may be able to help with shopping or gardening, children

with household chores, and partners with getting you dressed. You will be much better company for those around you! Plan ahead and work out what you need and who your helpers are.

Learn as much as you can about your condition and how it can be managed. Get to know the health professionals who can help and call them when you need to. Many rheumatology departments and charities have telephone helplines.

Community services can advise you on home adaptations or financial support. They may be able to organize help for you with your shopping or personal care.

Look for a local self-management programme for people who have long-term medical conditions. This gives people the opportunity to support each other and swap tips. Ask your family doctor for details.

HELPLINES
Various support services and rheumatology departments have set up helplines that you can contact for advice.

Coping with pain

People with arthritis usually have mild to moderate pain, stiffness, and inflammation in their joints. From time to time, these symptoms flare up and make the arthritis feel much worse. Flare-ups may be attributable to excessive use of the joints, but are often bewilderingly inexplicable and unpredictable, causing a great deal of anxiety. When healthcare professionals are not on hand to treat your flare-ups, you can turn to some simple, safe, and effective means for coping with your pain and managing your arthritis. These remedies can also reduce inflammation and stiffness, and improve your quality of life.

Reducing pain helps you regain control of your independence and manage your arthritis better.

What causes pain?

Pain is the response of the nervous system when an injury or disease damages the tissues of the body. It is often thought of as a simple alarm system that stimulates the body to take protective action to avoid additional damage. However, as anyone who regularly feels pain will tell you, there are types of persistent (chronic) pain that defy all reason and seem to serve no purpose whatsoever.

The type of pain depends on the person who is experiencing it as well as on its cause. Different people are likely to feel pain in different ways. Some have a low threshold and feel low levels of pain more acutely than others who seem able to withstand intense pain without complaint. Mood and personality can also determine the way you feel pain – stress, fear, and anxiety can make pain feel worse.

The pain gate

How the pain response mechanism actually works is something of a mystery. One explanation, called the pain gate theory, can help to visualize the effects of pain and its management.

According to the theory, there is a pain gate through which nervous impulses carrying the message of pain must pass. Normally, the gate is closed but when a pain severe enough – for example, in a flare-up that irritates the nerves in the skin, joints, and muscles – the nervous impulses pass through the gate and reach the brain where the pain is registered and interpreted.

Various remedies have the effect of shutting – or at least partly blocking – the pain gate. On the other hand, stress and anxiety can open the gate or make it easier for the nerve impulses to pass through.

Relieving pain

The body has its own way of relieving pain, at least for short periods. The brain and spinal cord produce endorphins and encephalins that belong to the same chemical family as morphine and have a similar sedative effect.

Treating pain

Flare-ups affect many people with chronic and fluctuating conditions, particularly rheumatoid arthritis but also osteoarthritis. They can last for weeks or months before they subside and better days return.

There are a number of different ways of treating pain when it flares up. Doctors usually prescribe drugs and occupational therapists, physical therapists, nurses, and podiatrists (who treat feet) use various kinds of intervention.

However, it is a good idea to discover ways of coping with your own unique pain. Then, when your symptoms of pain, swelling, and inflammation flare up, you are not so reliant on seeing your doctor or healthcare professional and have your own way of managing your symptoms.

Ways to reduce pain

Reducing pain helps you regain control of your independence and manage your arthritis better. There are a number of ways you can choose to reduce your pain, such as massage, applying heat or cold, and breathing and relaxation exercises. You may also find that they make your pain-relieving medication work better.

Some remedies work by releasing naturally occurring endorphins while others reduce your muscle tension, which helps decrease pain and improves the blood supply to muscles to enable freer movement.

Heat and cold

People with arthritis often turn to applying heat and cold to a joint to control the pain of a flare-up (see p.148). Sensations of heat and cold increase the number of nerve impulses that block pain signals and shut the pain gate. In addition, heat is a particularly

PRACTICAL TIPS

MANAGING FLARE-UPS

● Rest, but not in bed. Avoid or reduce activities that aggravate your pain – for example, prolonged standing or walking – for a couple of days until the pain subsides.

● Use heat or cold – or whatever you find eases your pain – several times each day (see p.148).

● If you feel anxious and tense, practise deep breathing and relaxation techniques (see p.150 and p.151) to help you calm down.

● Resume exercising gently once the pain starts to settle. If you do not move, your joints will stiffen up and your muscles will weaken and tire quickly.

● Re-establish your action plan (see p.73) and increase your activity levels gradually.

PRACTICAL TIPS

APPLYING HEAT OR COLD

● Lie down in a comfortable position and relax before applying either heat or cold.

● To apply heat, place a heat pack or a hot-water bottle wrapped in a towel on the painful, inflamed joint for 10–15 minutes.

● Remove the pack and gently move your joint. The combination of movement and rest is very important for pain relief.

● Replace the heat pack on the joint for another 5–10 minutes.

● To apply cold, place a cool pack or a bag of frozen peas wrapped in a towel on the painful, inflamed joint for 10–15 minutes. After removing the pack, move your joint gently to aid the pain relief.

good way of relaxing tense and aching muscles. Both heat and cold can improve your blood supply, reduce swelling, and enable you to move around more freely.

Warmth created by commercially available heat packs, a hot-water bottle wrapped in a towel, taking a hot bath, and wearing thermal clothing or bandages can reduce pain considerably.

Cooling can be produced with commercially available cool packs, coolant sprays, or a bag of frozen peas wrapped in a towel.

For most people, warming or cooling a joint is a safe technique. However, people who have circulatory problems should consult their doctor, physical therapist, or nurse. Make sure you don't burn your skin with a heat pack or hot-water bottle. Whatever method you use, avoid becoming uncomfortably hot or cold.

Massage

Massage and rubbing a painful body part relieves muscle tension, improves circulation, and disperses the fluid in swollen joints and muscles. It is a natural reaction to pain. Massage and rubbing effectively shuts the pain gate by stimulating the nerves in the skin, muscles, and joints, thereby blocking pain signals.

The physical contact in massage has been shown to be profoundly comforting, probably by releasing endorphins and encephalins, which reduce heart and breathing rates. Some of the pain relief from moisturizers, lotions, oils, gels, and creams is probably due to the massage needed to apply them.

Gently massaging painful joints or muscles for 5–10 minutes is a very effective, safe, and pleasurable way to relieve pain.

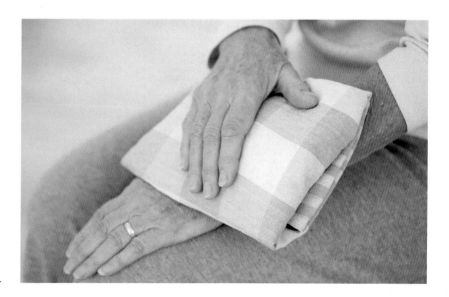

FROZEN PEAS
The cool temperature of a bag of frozen peas wrapped in a towel can relieve pain, improve the blood supply, and reduce swelling.

Water therapy

For thousands of years, people have used water therapy to treat arthritic conditions. Water therapy relieves pain by using the warmth and buoyancy of water to relax your muscles and reduce the weight-bearing load and stress on your legs and trunk.

Spa therapy

This residential treatment involves bathing in naturally heated water, which is often rich in minerals, and applying hot mud packs. These are combined with the psychological benefits of receiving respite care and gentle movement.

The effectiveness of spa therapy lies, at least in part, to the absence of domestic pressures, the relaxing environment, and a holistic health approach. However, it is expensive and has limited availability.

Hydrotherapy

This form of spa therapy uses the buoyancy, assistance, and resistance properties of warm water to help you exercise more effectively. It does not use mud packs or a holistic approach.

Hydrotherapy is a very popular treatment and is cheaper than spa therapy. However, it still requires dedicated facilities and therapists. Limited healthcare budgets mean that only a minority of people receive hydrotherapy – and most only have a brief, one-off course.

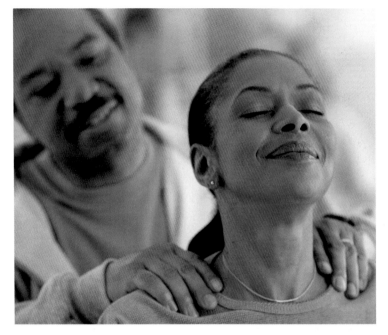

Aquatherapy

A growing number of community pools run aquatherapy classes that offer most of the benefits of hydrotherapy. They provide you with the opportunity to participate in controlled water-based exercises while supervised by experienced therapists at a moderate cost. If you cannot find an aquatherapy class, exercise gently in your local swimming pool to keep your stiff and painful joints moving.

Electrical stimulation

Transcutaneous electrical neuromuscular stimulation (TENS) is a non-invasive treatment for pain control that may work by shutting the pain gate. It may also stimulate the release of endorphins

MASSAGE
The healing power of touch means that massage brings relaxation and calm to tense muscles and painful joints.

Water therapy relieves pain by using the warmth and buoyancy of water to relax muscles and reduce the weight-bearing load and stress on your legs and trunk.

and encephalins, which help to relieve your pain, relax your tense muscles, and slow your breathing.

Physical therapists use several pieces of electrical equipment to reduce pain, but the best scientific evidence supports TENS as being the most effective.

TENS machines are readily available at modest cost and for home use. Consult your doctor before using a TENS machine and ask a physiotherapist to show you how to use it.

A TENS machine is a safe way of relieving pain. It delivers small electrical pulses that pass through electrodes taped to the skin where you are feeling pain. You can use it for about an hour or so, whether you are sitting, standing, or gently moving around.

There are some important safety concerns when using a TENS machine. Don't use one if you are pregnant (except for relieving pain during labour), nor if you have a pacemaker or heart condition. Never place the electrodes of a TENS machine near the carotid artery in your neck.

Relaxation and breathing

When you are in pain you start to think the worst of everything. You become stressed, exacerbating your negative thoughts (see p.154) and increasing your feeling of

being helplessly controlled by pain. This vicious circle needs to be broken so that you can begin to regain control.

The first step is to recognize the signs of increased stress, tension, and anxiety. These include shallow breathing, feeling uptight, and being nervous.

Notice how situations that make you stressed and anxious increase the muscle tension in your neck, shoulders, back, and legs. Notice, too, how these feelings are associated with pain. Try to avoid such situations and learn some techniques that help you relax, feel happier, and sleep better.

Two quick exercises

Many relaxation techniques can help to reduce tension and anxiety. The most common involve deep breathing and exercises that contract and relax your muscles in a progressive way.

There are two quick exercises that you can practise almost any time, any place, anywhere (see Deep Breathing, left, and Muscle Relaxation, p.151). Practise them when you are not stressed so that you can become more confident in your ability.

At first you may be sceptical that such simple techniques will help you control pain, but try them and see. If they don't work, at least you can say you have tried and will have lost little. If they work, you will gain a great deal.

PRACTICAL TIPS

DEEP BREATHING

● Sit or stand up straight without forcefully breathing. Gently breathe in, allowing your chest to expand fully.

● Relax your shoulders.

● Place a hand on your abdomen just below your ribcage.

● Take a slow, deep breath in through your nose and feel your hand and stomach rising up.

● When your lungs are fully expanded, slowly breathe out through your mouth – feel your abdomen and hand gently sink.

● Repeat this for four or five deep breaths, then rest and breathe in a normal relaxed way for a couple of minutes. If necessary, repeat the exercise for 5–10 minutes.

Alternating activity with rest

Physical activity is unquestionably good for controlling arthritic pain, but so, too, are rest and relaxation. Try to avoid getting tired because it leads to muscle weakness, which increases the risk of further pain and joint damage.

Most people begin to experience pain after doing an activity for a relatively short time. But they often continue with the task until it is completed or pain becomes so bad they are forced to rest.

Periods of rest

A better solution is to limit the time you spend doing the activity by interspersing it with periods of rest. This alternation of rest and activity will allow you to continue your everyday life within bearable limits of pain and discomfort.

First identify the activities that cause you pain and think about the way you are doing them. Find out how long each activity takes to start making you feel tired or to have some mild discomfort, then take a short rest.

For example, if you start to feel some discomfort after a 20-minute stint of gardening, rest for 5–10 minutes, then return to the task. Take another break if pain starts to increase again or finish the task another time.

If you record your activity–rest times you will find the activity time increases before you need to rest, and the activity becomes much easier with much less pain.

PRACTICAL TIPS

MUSCLE RELAXATION

● Stop whatever activity you are doing. Stand, sit, or (preferably) lie down somewhere quiet.

● Take a few deep breaths. If you're anxious your breathing will be quick and shallow, which will make you uptight.

● Close your eyes and imagine a relaxing scene, such as sitting on a quiet beach on a sunny day.

● Starting from your shoulders, tighten your muscles, hold them tight for 5 seconds, then relax.

● Feel the tension release from your muscles and joints. They will feel looser and make you feel lighter. Work through each muscle group, from the top of your body to your toes.

● Hold on to that feeling of relaxation for 30 seconds before returning to the activity you were doing.

RELAXATION
One of the best ways to cope with your pain is relaxation – it relieves tense muscles, calms you down, and gives you back control.

Coping with stress

Living with the ups and downs of arthritis can disturb your emotional state so that you feel frustration, anger, guilt, sadness, loss, fear, anxiety, or hurt. At times, it can be an emotional roller-coaster, especially when you are diagnosed or during periods of yet more pain, fatigue, or uncertainty about your treatment or the future. Emotional changes can increase your levels of stress while your negative thoughts and beliefs can fuel the vicious cycle of pain, fatigue, and stress. Psychological ways of managing stress can break this cycle, reducing your pain and fatigue, and helping to make you happier.

Whatever the situation, you can choose how you wish to react to it because you have a measure of free will.

What is stress?

Stress is a part of life. You can feel it in the painful, anxious, exciting, depressing, irritating, dangerous, or frightening experiences that affect us all every single day.

Stress is also the way your body and mind respond to each of these stressors – chemically in the way your nerves work, physically in the way your body responds, and psychologically in the way your mind reacts (see The Body's Reaction to Stress, opposite).

Sources of stress can be found in changes to your lifestyle (such as work, family, finances, home,

and friends), imagined changes (such as fears about the future or your inability to do things), and everyday hassles (such as traffic jams, queues, noise, problems at work, and bad news). The effects and symptoms of arthritis are also a source of stress. Stress itself also increases the symptoms of arthritis.

When faced with a potential stressor you wonder if you can cope. If you believe you can, your stress response is less likely to be activated. If you believe you can't, or are faced with too many worries and physical problems, you are more likely to be stressed and emotionally upset.

Changing your responses to stress

You need to release stress before it builds up and starts to dominate your life. Many methods can help relieve stress, including exercise, movement therapies, relaxation, breathing, and meditation.

The mind is also a powerful tool in dealing with stress. One of the advantages of using psychological approaches to stress is that you can be in control of what happens inside your own mind. Whatever the situation, you can choose how you wish to react to it because you have a measure of free will. Our attitudes, thoughts, and beliefs shape our responses to stress – not events, past or present. Changing the way you think takes work and mental effort, especially if you have been under stress for a long time. However, with perseverance the rewards are a happier outlook in life and better health.

The ABC method

Cognitive therapists and life coaches, who can help us unravel and understand the mental knots and confused thinking that affect us all, have developed very

TALKING HELPS
The stress of some situations and thoughts can be eased simply by talking them through with a person who cares for you.

THE BODY'S REACTION TO STRESS

When you are stressed, a range of chemical, physical, and psychological changes occur within you. Many of the physical and psychological changes are like the symptoms you may experience as you cope with the pain and inflammation of arthritis. It is important to recognize stress and realize that it can contribute to some of your pain, fatigue, muscle tension, and sleep problems. Stress management techniques can reduce these symptoms and help you to cope with your arthritis.

CHEMICAL CHANGES

- The body produces higher levels of three hormones – adrenaline, noradrenaline, and cortisol. These increase heart rate, blood pressure, respiration, and metabolism, and lead to the release of chemicals that control the functions of the body's systems.

- The brain produces less of the hormone serotonin, thereby causing sleep disturbance.

PHYSICAL CHANGES

- Breathing becomes faster and shallower
- Tense muscles
- Heart rate quickens
- Skin may be clammy

If stress levels stay high:
- Increased fatigue, aches, and pains
- Stomach and bowel disturbances
- Headaches
- Raised blood pressure
- Loss of appetite

PSYCHOLOGICAL CHANGES

- Increased worrying or irritability
- Increased depression
- Images of losing control and being helpless
- Poorer concentration and memory
- Poorer self-image, less self-belief
- Increased automatic negative thoughts
- Restlessness, accident proneness, poorer time management, lower productivity

What you want to develop is a logical, rational approach to dispute your thoughts.

effective strategies for coping with stress. One of these, the ABC method, may help you understand how you respond to a stressful event and how you can change your response. A is the Activating event, B represents the Beliefs and thoughts that are triggered in your mind, and C summarizes the Consequences – the emotional, physical, or behavioural changes.

When some event happens that triggers a stress response inside you, particularly when you have been under a lot of stress, there may be negative consequences. For instance, you get emotionally upset and your pain and fatigue get worse. This activating event seems to lead to the consequences – but is this really true? Perhaps the event is the last straw and that other, more deep-seated problems are causing the consequences.

Identify negative thoughts

The first step to changing the nature of your stress response is to identify the beliefs and thoughts that run through your mind.

As we become progressively stressed, we get more emotionally upset and are likely to think more and more automatic negative thoughts (ANTs). These are called automatic because the negative thoughts just pop into our minds involuntarily and, at the time, are very believable.

The higher your stress levels, the more you believe these ANTs are true. They run through your mind and become difficult to shift. They trigger more negative thoughts and increase your stress response still further. ANTs can become a habit, like thinking traps you fall into time and again.

However, once you start to identify your ANTs, you can start changing them. Be honest with yourself about the thinking traps you can fall into – for example:
- All or nothing thinking – you see things in extremes.
- Mind reading – you know what others are thinking without first hearing what they have to say.
- Personalization – you blame yourself for events that are not your responsibility.
- Emotional reasoning – you feel something strongly therefore it must be true.
- Labelling – you often attach a negative label to an event.

TRAFFIC JAMS
One of the most irritating sources of stress is a traffic jam – it very rarely fails to trigger a negative response that leaves us feeling tense and anxious.

USING A THOUGHT AND SYMPTOM DIARY (THE ABCDE METHOD)

Keep a diary that records the dates and activating events that trigger stress. Fill it in as soon as you can while the event is fresh in your mind. Record your thoughts, beliefs, emotions, and the consequences. Then compose your disputing thoughts that put a positive spin on the event and the effective actions to take next time. In this example, a woman with rheumatoid arthritis feels stress because her two boys won't put on their coats for school and end up rushing to catch the bus.

BELIEFS/THOUGHTS	CONSEQUENCES	DISPUTING THOUGHTS	EFFECTIVE ACTIONS
• "I'll never get them to school on time." • "I'm such an awful mother!" • "I can never cope with these kids, I'm useless!" • "Every morning is one long struggle!"	• Feel frustrated, hassled. Tense muscles. Tired. • Shallow breathing, heart racing, feel stressed. • Later in day, pain and fatigue worse. Headache. Worrying. • Difficult managing so many jobs.	• "Most of the time we manage to get to the bus on time." • "Being a bit late sometimes is OK." • "I can cope with the kids. In fact, most of the time I do cope."	• Take deep breaths. • Give them a kiss – the boys always want to get away then! • Get lunch ready the night before to avoid rushing in the morning. • Talk to the boys about why I need them to help.

• Discounting the positive – you see things negatively and push aside any positive experiences or personal qualities that you have.

• Fortune-telling – you believe you have the power to predict the future accurately.

• Musts and shoulds – you steadfastly abide by internal rules that cannot be broken.

Develop an effective outlook

The next step in changing the way you think is to build on your ABC. Add a D and an E by Disputing your negative thoughts and beliefs, then develop an Effective outlook.

In hindsight, we look back at negative thoughts and rationally think "Of course, I see now that isn't true." What you want to develop is a logical, rational approach to dispute your thoughts and avoid the consequences at the time of the stressful event, to stop yourself sliding into emotional distress. Such an approach will help to train your mind to have a more positive, flexible, resilient, and effective outlook, so that you are better able to cope with stress-triggering events in the future.

Keep a thought and symptom diary (see above) to help you focus on the various aspects of the ABCDE model and to complete the process of changing the way you think. Once you have identified your negative thoughts, start disputing them. Try the following:

• What is the evidence for the thoughts you are thinking?

• Are you applying double standards to yourself?

MEDITATION
One of the best ways to quieten your mind and relax the body is to practise meditation every day.

KEEPING A JOURNAL
Here are some ideas to write in your journal:

● A thought and symptom diary (see p.155) to help you see the link between thoughts, feelings, stress, and worsening arthritis symptoms. Keep track of your disputing thoughts and other coping ideas.

● Problem-solving for practical solutions.

● Records of exercises and activities.

● Effectiveness of drugs, complementary therapies, and diet.

● Keep a record of how well you sleep and how often you wake at night.

● Goal-setting (see p.73).

● Think in shades of grey instead of in all or nothing terms. Give different aspects of an event a score on a scale of 0–100.
● Why are you calling yourself names for failing at something?
● Change the musts and shoulds and ease up on yourself.
● List the pros and cons of your negative thought, feeling, or behaviour. This is good for developing a rational perspective.
● Develop positive statements and find inspirational sayings to write on cards (keep them in your pocket, bag, or on the fridge door to remind you) or in a journal. Read these to affirm to yourself your abilities and positive actions.
● Use other coping strategies that will help, such as deep breathing techniques (see p.150), relaxation training (see pp.150–151), and the planning ahead principles in joint protection (see p.176).

Mind–body exercises

Meditation, deep breathing (see p.150), and visualization (see p.157), are effective for reducing stress. They can help to restore a more balanced outlook on life, reduce tension, and lower blood pressure. Practise them regularly – every day would be best.

Meditation

This mind–body technique is an excellent way to create a relaxed state of awareness. Meditation helps you to develop calmness, improve your concentration, and relieve pain, stress, and depression. Try the following sequence:

Find the right time, such as the morning or before bed. You will develop skills more quickly if you practise regularly. Start for just 5 or 10 minutes, a few times a week. Find the right place – a quiet special place where there are no interruptions and where the room is warm. Personalize it with a meditation object you like – for example, a candle, a favourite stone, a remarkable fir cone, a beautiful flower, or an appealing painting. Burn incense and play soothing music if you wish.

Sit down or lie comfortably. Support your head and keep your back straight so you can breathe freely and deeply. Wearing loose clothes will help, too.

Quieten your body with deep breathing. Focus on your special meditation object (either in reality or in your mind) as your focal point. Don't try too hard. Let your feelings and thoughts drift in and out of your consciousness without becoming involved in them.

Gradually imagine the feelings and thoughts are like ripples in a pond, moving away from you.

Stay focused on your breathing. If you become distracted, don't worry – just bring your attention back to your focal point. Whatever you feel – peaceful, bored, or tense – is normal. It takes time to develop inner stillness. As you practise regularly, so you will find that it becomes easier.

When you feel calmer, centre your mind on the word "peace". Meditate on this word and let it fill both your mind and body.

After a few minutes, release the word "peace" so that only the essence of peace remains within you. Notice how relaxed you feel. Breathe deeply and gradually focus your mind back to the room.

Give yourself time to persevere with meditation. Before long it will grow more and more effective.

VISUALIZATION

This mind–body exercise can be a powerful way of relaxing. It is also called guided imagery because you guide yourself through a relaxing scene and let your troubles ebb away.

A number of visualization CDs are available – try to find one you like, then sit or lie comfortably with your arms and legs relaxed.

Alternatively, you could devise your own sequence and either record and listen to it, or learn it and repeat it to yourself. The following excerpt from a sequence may inspire you:

"Breathe deeply through your nose and exhale slowly through your mouth. Again, take a deep breath in slowly...and slowly exhale...feel your tension melt away...your body feels heavy and warm...listen to your heart beat.

"Imagine you are on a warm beach, by a quiet calm sea...as the water gently laps, inhale and exhale...one after the other your negative emotions ebb away...like the waves on the sand...worries... frustration...pain...sadness...ebb away. You're content...at peace... relaxed...happier...lighter..."

When you're ready, end the exercise by wiggling your fingers and toes, and return to the every day feeling refreshed.

RELAXING SCENE
A good focus for visualization is a gentle scene where waves break rhythmically on a sandy shore.

Maintaining your mobility

Arthritis can limit your ability to do things and so you may be tempted, even encouraged, to rest and become less active. Although this is understandable, it would be a mistake because you would start to lose your mobility and your flexibility. All the activities you enjoy, such as walking, dancing, swimming, or cycling, can become hard to do. The exercises that follow will help you to maintain and improve your mobility so that you can manage your arthritis more effectively.

Follow the exercise routine

Before you start, read the Ten Exercise Rules (see p.159). The first rule is the most important: whatever exercise you do, make sure you are stable and safe. Always have something solid to grab on to but make sure it will also support you.

In the exercises on the following pages, the head turns, head rolls, sit-to-stands, step-ups, and squats, can make you feel dizzy, so be very careful. If possible, do them with someone beside you. You can either do every exercise as part of a daily plan or focus on individual exercises according to your needs.

Start with low-impact exercises that do not involve your bearing any weight. These are the ones in which you sit or lie on the floor or on a bed. Then build up to doing the weight-bearing exercises and functional activities, such as walking (see p.70).

Two groups of exercises

The exercises in this chapter can be classified into two groups. First are the flexibility exercises, which use minimal resistance to increase or maintain the range of movement of your joints.

Q&A

How can I tell if I have done too much exercise?

It is normal for your muscles to feel a bit stretched but they shouldn't ache too much. If after exercising you feel exhausted or your discomfort is worse than before then you have probably overdone it. Another telltale sign is if you are still sore or aching an hour after exercise. Perhaps more serious is when the pain, discomfort, or swelling lasts for a couple of days, or wakes you at night.

The second group of exercises uses a resistance (such as an elastic band or your body weight) to increase strength.

In both these types of exercise, try to "nudge the boundaries" of your capabilities, challenging yourself to gently, gradually move a little further or work a little harder. Once you have reached a level you are content with, keep that level of exercise going to maintain the gains you have achieved. If you continually do less and less you will slip back and lose mobility.

Performing the exercises well, with controlled movement, is as important as repeating the exercise more often or for longer. In addition, try to hold the position at the end of a range-of-movement exercise, such as the shoulder rotation, so that you feel a gentle stretch. Keep your breathing relaxed as you do this because

it increases the effectiveness of the stretch and maximizes your effort. Being too forceful and enthusiastic or "aggressive" can increase pain and discomfort.

Adapt the guidelines

In the exercises that follow, the instructions suggest how long you could hold a particular movement for and how many repetitions of an exercise you can do – but these are just guidelines. Some people may be able to do more right from the start, others less.

Adapt the guidelines to suit you, but be careful if you are not used to exercising: what seems like a simple and easy task can cause discomfort and pain, which may lead to anxiety that you have caused damage by doing too much. Err on the side of caution – start gently and increase gradually.

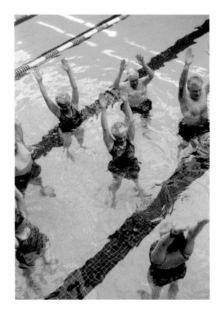

WATER EXERCISE
Warm-water swimming pools are good places to exercise many of your joints and improve their mobility and flexibility.

PRACTICAL TIPS

TEN EXERCISE RULES

● When doing an exercise always ensure you're stable and safe. For example, if you stand, have something near to hold on to.

● Start each new exercise gently and cautiously.

● Increase the amount or kind of exercise gradually over days and weeks.

● Work hard but don't cause prolonged pain or discomfort.

● Rest on days when your joints are painful. When the pain subsides, resume exercising gently.

● Perform the exercises using well-controlled movement – quality is as important as quantity.

● Set yourself realistic goals.

● Write an action plan and tell people your goals.

● Pace yourself – little and often is just as good as one strenuous session.

● Understand that exercise does not cure arthritis and episodes of pain are not related to exercising.

Neck exercises

Head turns and head rolls are two simple neck exercises that you can practise regularly to improve the movement of your head on your shoulders. Before you start, make sure you are standing – or sitting – straight and tall. Imagine a string, connected to the crown at the top of your head, is holding you up and extending your neck. Keep your shoulders and upper limbs relaxed at all times. Breathe in through your nose and out through your mouth, slowly and gently.

HEAD TURNS

Keep your shoulders relaxed.

Keep your head upright and try to stop your head tilting to the side as you turn.

Slowly turn your head to look over your right shoulder without tilting it to the side. Feel a gentle stretch and tightness in your neck. Breathe gently. Hold the position for 5 or 6 seconds.

As you turn your head, feel a gentle stretch and tightness in your neck.

You can do this head-turning exercise either sitting or standing. If you are standing, make sure you are next to a wall or something to grab on to just in case you feel dizzy.

Now turn to look over your left shoulder, again without tilting your head to the side. Hold the position for 5 or 6 seconds. Repeat the full exercise sequence 5 or 6 times.

HEAD ROLLS

Make sure your shoulders are relaxed.

Start with your shoulders relaxed and your eyes looking forwards. Slowly let your head fall to the front so that your chin drops down towards your chest and you are looking at the floor.

Slowly roll your head to the left. As you do so, bring your left ear as close to your left shoulder as you comfortably can, with your eyes looking in the direction your head is moving.

Continue to move your head in a wide circle, from left to right. When you reach midway, look upwards towards the ceiling and feel a gentle stretch in the muscles in the front of your neck.

Keep your eyes looking in the direction your head is moving.

Come down with your right ear as close to your right shoulder as you comfortably can. Relax. Repeat 3 or 4 circles. Repeat the whole sequence, this time circling to the right.

Shoulder exercises

These three exercises are excellent for improving the range of movement in both your shoulders. The windmill is particularly good for helping the ball-and-socket joint in each shoulder reach their fullest extent in any direction.

Each of the exercises will strengthen the shoulder joints and the muscles surrounding them, which will help you cope better with everyday tasks such as putting on your clothes, brushing your hair, driving, cleaning, and gardening.

WINDMILLS

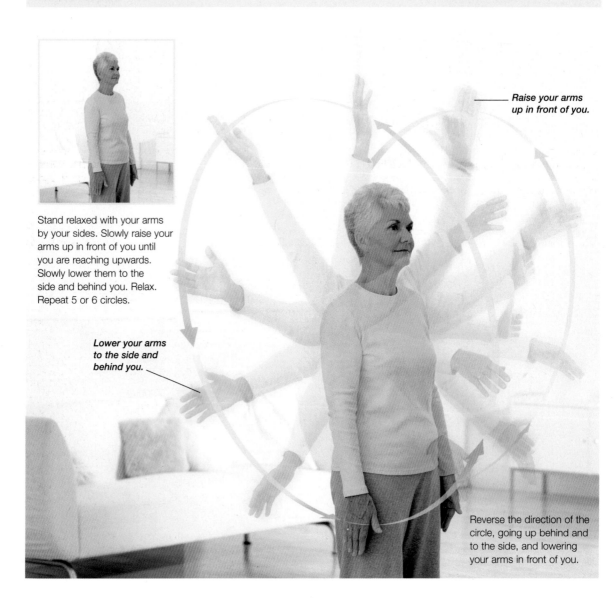

Stand relaxed with your arms by your sides. Slowly raise your arms up in front of you until you are reaching upwards. Slowly lower them to the side and behind you. Relax. Repeat 5 or 6 circles.

Raise your arms up in front of you.

Lower your arms to the side and behind you.

Reverse the direction of the circle, going up behind and to the side, and lowering your arms in front of you.

SHOULDER ROTATION

Clasp your hands behind your head, with your fingers interlocked. If you can't reach behind your head because it is uncomfortable, just place your hands as far back on the top of your head as you can. Gently push your elbows outwards – but only within your comfort zone. Feel a gentle stretch under your arms beneath the shoulders. Hold this position for 5 seconds if you can. Breathe out. Bring your forearms back close to your ears. Repeat the exercise 5 or 6 times.

"BACK DRY"

Roll up a small towel and grip it as if you were drying your back, placing your right arm over the top of your right shoulder and your left arm in the small of your back. With your left hand gently pull the towel down, feeling a gentle pull in your right arm. Hold for 5 or 6 seconds. Now pull the towel up with your right hand and feel a gentle pull in your left arm. Hold for 5 or 6 seconds. Repeat the exercise 10 times. Then swap your hands – the left above your left shoulder and your right in the small of your back.

Back exercises

The sit-ups and easy press-ups are two of the many exercises that can help you with the flexibility of your lower back. If you have a pain in your lower back, consult your doctor or physiotherapist before trying these exercises.

Both exercises involve you lying down – if you use the floor, spread out a mat or towel to make it a little more comfortable. If you have difficulty bending down, take time to get into position and relax for a few minutes before starting.

SIT-UPS

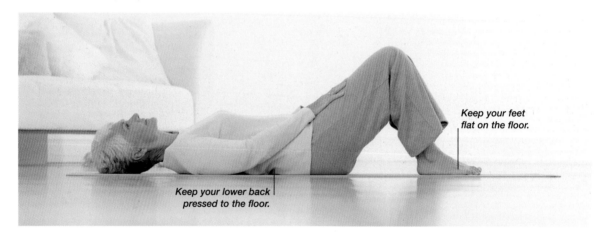

Keep your feet flat on the floor.

Keep your lower back pressed to the floor.

This exercise is designed to strengthen the muscles in your abdomen, which are important for the mobility of your back. Lie down on your back on the floor (or on a bed) with your knees bent and place your hands on your thighs. Relax your shoulders and let them sink towards the floor. Become conscious of your breathing as you inhale and exhale from your abdomen.

Don't try to reach too far with your hands.

Don't try to raise your head and shoulders too far above the floor.

Slowly run your hands up your thighs towards your knees, gently raising your head and shoulders off the floor. Don't reach too far. If you can, hold the position for 5 or 6 seconds, then breathe out. Relax as you roll down slowly. Rest for 5 or 6 seconds. Repeat the exercise 5 or 6 times. Over a few weeks increase the number of sit-ups and hold them for a little bit longer.

EASY PRESS-UPS

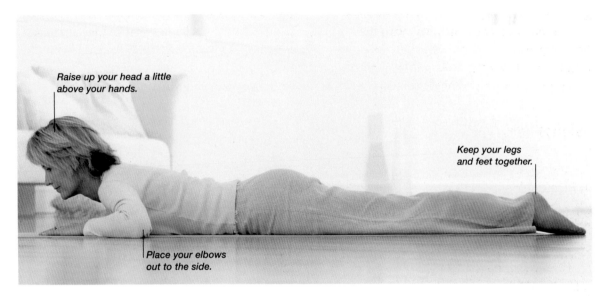

Raise up your head a little above your hands.

Keep your legs and feet together.

Place your elbows out to the side.

This exercise increases the mobility of the spine in your lower back and also the sacroiliac joints where the spine meets the pelvis. Lie face down on a mat or towel on the floor, with your elbows pointing out to the side and your hands placed flat on the floor under your shoulders. Relax your whole body and breathe gently. Raise up your head.

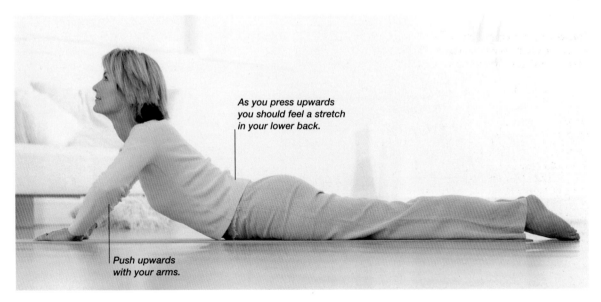

As you press upwards you should feel a stretch in your lower back.

Push upwards with your arms.

Inhale and hold in your breath as you push up with your arms and slowly straighten your elbows. Lift up your head and shoulders as high as you can within your comfort zone. Look up at the ceiling and, as you feel a stretch in the region of your lower back, breathe out. Feel your lower back sag slightly as you breathe out. Hold this position for 5 or 6 seconds. Let your arms relax as they allow the trunk of your body to lower slowly to the floor. Repeat the exercise 5 or 6 times.

Leg and hip exercises

The following exercises will help people with arthritis to improve and maintain the mobility in their hips and knees. They help to ease any stiffness you might feel and build up strength in the muscles surrounding the joints.

People with osteoarthritis of the knee or hip should find particular benefit from the step-ups and the sit-to-stand exercises. Make sure you always work within your comfort zone and avoid overstretching yourself.

STEP-UPS

Keep your head still and look ahead.

Hold on to give yourself support.

Raise your left leg and step up.

Step up and down with your right foot.

Place your left foot on a low, stable step (e.g. on the bottom stair or on a pile of 3 telephone directories). Hold on to the wall, banisters, or chair for support. Keeping your left foot on the step, step up and down with your right foot for a minute. Repeat 5 or 6 times, resting for a short time between each. Put your right foot on the step and repeat the exercise. As you gradually increase the number of step-ups, raise the height of the step (ensuring you are stable and safe) to a maximum of about 45cm.

GENTLE SQUATS

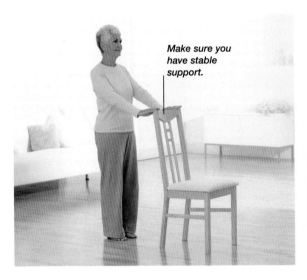

Make sure you have stable support.

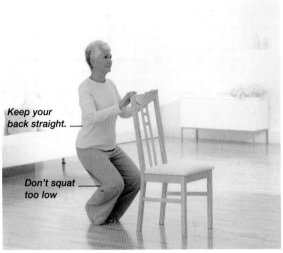

Keep your back straight.

Don't squat too low

Stand upright with your feet flat on the floor and your gaze looking straight ahead. Gently steady yourself by resting your hands on a stable object (such as the back of a chair) positioned in front of you. Keeping your back straight, slowly bend your knees into a gentle squat and then straighten your knees until you are standing again. Repeat 10 times. As you improve, squat down a little further, but not beyond 90 degrees, and never squat fully as it puts great strain on your knees.

HIP ROTATIONS

Turn your foot inwards.

Turn your foot outwards.

Stand upright with one hand resting on a stable object, such as the back of a chair. Place your right hand on the front of your right hip and hitch up the hip so that your right foot is 2–3cm off the ground. Turn your foot inwards to the left as far as it will go (feel your hip turning inwards under your hand). Hold the position for 5 or 6 seconds. Turn your foot outwards to the right (again feeling your hip turn) and hold for 5 or 6 seconds. Repeat the sequence 10 times. Then repeat with the left foot 10 times.

LEG STRENGTHENING

Tie an elastic inner tube of a bicycle tyre or a commercially available resistive exercise band to an immovable object, such as the leg of a chair. Loop it around your right foot.

Sit upright with your back straight and your head still.

Sit upright on the chair and slowly straighten your knee as far as you can, stretching the band. Hold the position for 5 seconds. Let the tension in the band slowly pull your leg back to the starting position. Repeat for 1–2 minutes. Then repeat using your left foot.

As you improve, perform the exercise for longer, hold your leg straight for longer, and/or increase the resistance by making the loop smaller or using a stiffer resistive band.

Tie the elastic band to a chair leg and loop it around your foot.

SIT-TO-STANDS

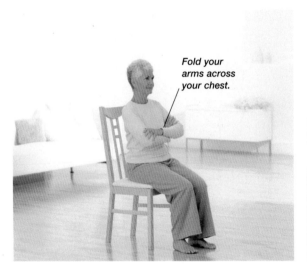

Fold your arms across your chest.

Remain standing for a few seconds.

Sit upright on a chair, with your gaze straight ahead, your feet flat on the ground, and your arms folded across your chest. Stand up slowly without using your arms and remain in the standing position for a few seconds. Sit down slowly. Continue to do these sit-to-stands for about a minute. Over a period of a few weeks, try to increase the number of sit-to-stands you do – or start from a lower chair or the next-to-bottom stair. Never strain yourself and always make sure you are in control.

KNEE FLEXIONS

Look straight ahead.

Keep your neck vertical.

You should feel a comfortable stretch in your leg.

Hold position for 5–6 seconds.

Sit on the floor or bed with your legs together and stretched out in front of you. Place your hands on the floor behind you so that they take the weight of your upper body. Keep your neck vertical and your gaze straight ahead.

Slowly move your right knee towards you until it is bent and you can feel a comfortable stretch. Hold this position for 5 or 6 seconds before straightening your leg again. Rest for 3 seconds. Repeat the sequence 10 times. Repeat using your left leg.

TRUNK ROTATIONS

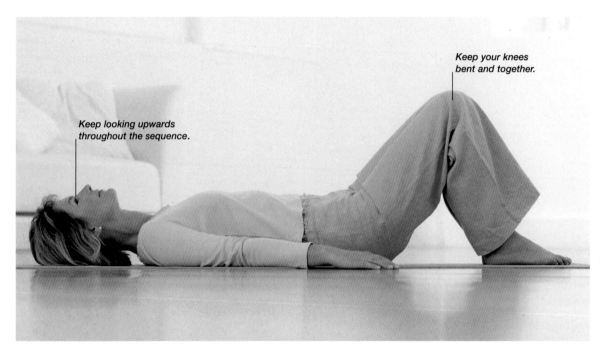

Keep looking upwards throughout the sequence.

Keep your knees bent and together.

Lie on the floor or a bed with knees bent, shoulders relaxed, arms beside you, and looking upwards. Slowly let your knees fall to the right, keeping them together as you do so and still looking up (below). Stop when you feel a gentle stretch in your lower back and left thigh, and hold the position for 5 or 6 seconds.

Return to the starting position. Now repeat the exercise, this time letting your knees fall gently to the left (below) and holding for 5 or 6 seconds. Repeat the whole sequence 10 times. Rest for 30 seconds. Repeat 5 times. Over a few weeks as your trunk loosens up, let your knees fall slightly further to the sides.

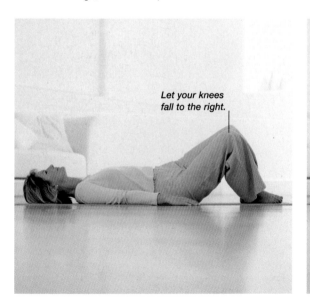

Let your knees fall to the right.

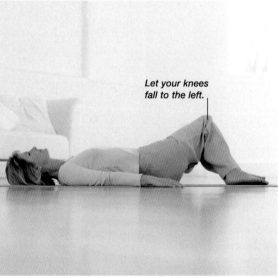

Let your knees fall to the left.

HIP EXTENSIONS

Keep your head still and looking at the floor.

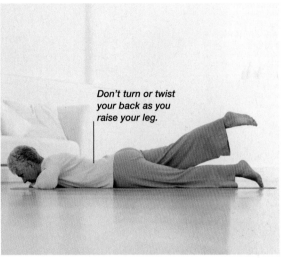

Don't turn or twist your back as you raise your leg.

Lie comfortably on your front on a mat on the floor (or on a bed) so you are resting your chin on your hands. Without turning or twisting your back, slowly raise your right leg up behind you about 7.5–10cm. Hold this position for 4 to 5 seconds if you can before slowly lowering your leg to the floor. Relax your body and breathe out. Repeat 5 times. Repeat with your left leg. As you improve, try to raise each leg a little higher, hold it up a little longer, and/or increase the number of leg raises.

HIP ABDUCTIONS

Use your hand on the floor to keep you stable.

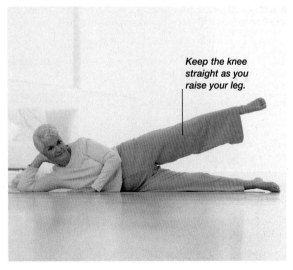

Keep the knee straight as you raise your leg.

Lie comfortably on your right side on a mat on the floor (or on a bed) and prop up your head with your right hand. Keeping your left knee straight, slowly raise your left leg into the air – about 60cm if you can. Hold the position for 5 or 6 seconds, then slowly lower the leg, and relax. Repeat 10 times. Turn over and repeat the exercise with your right leg. As you improve, increase the number of lifts, raise each leg a little higher, and hold it for a little longer. Make sure the movements are slow and controlled.

Protecting your joints

Joints and muscles have to last a lifetime, so taking care of them makes sense. Some of the ways of protecting your joints were developed in industry to reduce the strain on workers. You may already be doing some of them, while others can be hard to accept at first. Once you use the methods often enough in your daily life, you will reap the benefits. Less pain, less fatigue, and doing jobs more easily with less frustration will result – and you will have energy left over so you can enjoy life more.

Protecting your joints is not about giving up activities – just finding easier ways of doing them.

Why protect your joints?

How you stand and move your body affects the stress and strain you place upon your joints. For example, a slouched posture increases the stress on your back and neck. You will put strain on your muscles and joints if you repeat the same movement over and over, or if you hold a joint in the same restricted position for too long. Even using too much effort to do a job can be stressful.

We all develop movement habits that may not be the most efficient. But when you have arthritis this inefficiency increases your fatigue and adds to your pain.

Straining joints that are swollen and painful can further weaken the support structures of the joints (the ligaments and joint capsules). In time, deformities may develop. Straining muscles increases fatigue.

If it hurts, change it

Protecting your joints is not about giving up activities – just finding easier ways of doing them. Most people develop their own ways to reduce pain and fatigue over the years. But it takes time to work out solutions for yourself. People with arthritis often get used to pain, and medication can mask it, so you may not notice an activity causes strain, pain, or fatigue until afterwards. Then you regret overdoing it the next day. So the rule is: if it hurts, change it.

Shortcuts to making changes

The ideas in this chapter will help you take shortcuts to making the kind of changes that will keep your muscles and joints as healthy as possible. The sooner you make the changes, the better for your joints in the long run.

Making activities easier will not weaken your muscles – it will reduce your fatigue and pain, leaving you with more energy to exercise. The chapters on physical activity and mobility (see pp.64–73 and pp.158–171) show you how to move your joints fully and strengthen your muscles.

knuckles. Over time, this weakens ligaments and joints start to move in the direction of the pressure.

Look at how you move your joints and muscles during daily activities and see if you can find a way of doing them differently, applying the seven principles on p.174. Changing habits is tricky at first as the old ones kick in automatically. Once you get used to analysing what you are doing, the ideas will start to snowball.

A step-by-step technique

Start changing your habits in a step-by-step way. Pick a common daily activity, such as making a cup of tea. Watch how you use your hands and the joints and muscles that cause you pain.

Check to see how you hold your joints while moving and working. For example, are your wrists bent sideways or downwards rather

HOLDING A CUP
When you drink a cup of tea or coffee, try holding the cup with both hands rather than putting strain on the fingers of one hand.

Changing your habits

Arthritis can cause some joints to deform over time. For example, if you have rheumatoid arthritis your wrists can start to move downwards and your fingers point away from the thumb. In thumb osteoarthritis, a zig-zag shape can develop.

Many activities, such as lifting, can put a downward pressure or pull on the wrist. Others, such as opening a jar or turning taps, require twisting movements at the than in a straight line or upright? Is there hard pressure on the ends of your fingers and thumbs? Are you gripping too tightly?

If you answer yes to these questions, how can you change the movement or the activity to make it easier? Think about the seven principles to protect your joints (see below) and write down your solutions in a notebook. Practise this technique as often as you can over the next week or two.

Key principles to protect your joints

The following seven key principles use biomechanics and ergonomics to help you protect your joints and manage your fatigue:
● Use your larger, stronger muscles and joints.

● Avoid twisting actions.
● Spread the load over several of your joints.
● Use the least effort.
● Avoid staying in the same position for too long.
● Plan your activities more efficiently.
● Pace your activities.

Biomechanics is the use of efficient physical techniques for standing, sitting, walking, and bending, as well as lifting and handling objects. Ergonomics is the design of tasks and equipment to fit people's abilities to their activities and to their environment in the most effective way possible.

Use your larger, stronger muscles and joints

Don't put pressure on your small joints and muscles when your larger, stronger ones can do a job more effectively. For example, if you have hand problems you can carry bags over your forearm or shoulder (or use a backpack if you can). Another example is to use your thigh muscles and elbows to push up out of a chair rather than pushing down with your knuckles.

Avoid twisting actions

Twisting actions that use force can cause pain and discomfort. For example, rather than using your fingers to twist a tight lid off a jar, press down on it with the palm of the hand or hold the side of the jar lid between the curve of your

OPENING A JAR
The best way to unscrew the lid of a jar is to press down with your palm or hold the side of the jar lid between the curve of your thumb and fingers. Then unscrew the lid with your arm.

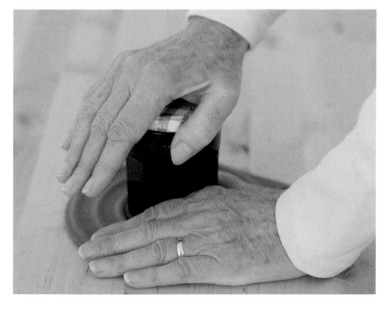

thumb and fingers. A small non-slip mat or a jar opener (available in kitchen shops) can also help.

If you have hip, knee, or foot problems, get up from a chair with your weight spread over both legs, rather than leaning to one side.

Spread the load over several of your joints

Don't rely on one joint to do a job when several joints can share the load. For example, use the palms of both hands to lift things. Try holding crockery and pots in both palms, rather than with fingers and thumbs – it also reduces the risk of dropping things.

When pouring water from a hot kettle, grip the handle with one hand while the palm of the other supports the side of the kettle with a cloth. Using two hands in this way cuts the strain on each wrist and hand by 50 per cent.

Use the least effort

The following ways will help you to minimize the effort you use to accomplish various tasks:

■ **DON'T GRIP OBJECTS TOO TIGHTLY**
If you have hand problems, use kitchen gadgets and household and DIY tools with non-slip handle surfaces so that you don't have to grip so hard. You can also pad out normal handles slightly – for example, with foam tubing from a DIY shop. To help you write, use a thicker pen or a pen grip (see p.139).

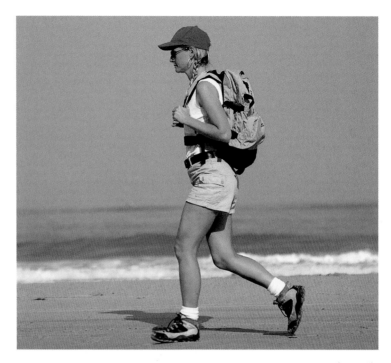

■ **USE WHEELS TO MOVE OBJECTS**
For example, use a plastic box trolley with an extending handle to move laundry round the house and garden, or to move the shopping from the car to the house. Use a briefcase with wheels and an extending handle to move your laptop and office papers.

■ **USE ASSISTIVE DEVICES** See p.140 for some of the many readily available assistive devices.

■ **USE LABOUR-SAVING EQUIPMENT**
Consider buying labour-saving household equipment, such as a tumble-drier and a dishwasher. The money is well spent if the equipment reduces your fatigue and pain, and gives you more energy and time to spend with your family and friends, and on activities you enjoy.

SPREAD THE LOAD
Using a backpack is a good example of spreading the load and letting the larger, stronger muscles take the strain.

TASK ANALYSIS: IRONING

Task analysis is a technique used in industry and management that can also help you with domestic jobs. It enables you to focus on ways of protecting your joints so that you do the job in hand with less stress and a minimum of effort. Ironing is an example of how you could use task analysis for a common household job.

PROBLEM	POSSIBLE SOLUTION
Amount of ironing	● Keep the amount of ironing to a minimum. Buy non-iron, easy-care, or tumble-dry items. Hang up clothes straight after drying to avoid creases. ● Ask yourself if you really need to iron the item.
Ironing board	● Leave the ironing board up (if room) or fix a drop-down board to a wall or buy a lightweight board. ● Use a board with a metal stand to lay the iron flat. Up-ending the iron strains your wrist. ● Use a reflective board cover so you don't have to iron both sides of an item.
Iron	● Fix a pull to the plug to get it in and out easily. ● Use a lightweight iron with a long flex, a good grip surface to the handle, and a flick switch to put steam function on and off.
Doing the ironing	● "Little and often" are the key watch words. ● Use an ironing stool to take the weight off your legs. Move around regularly. Take microbreaks. ● Wear a wrist splint. ● Keep the weight of the iron to a minimum – do the items that need steaming last so you just put water in when you need it.

Avoid staying in the same position for too long

Whenever you feel as though you're sitting or standing in the same position for a long time, change it. If you're in a sitting position, get up and move around for a minute or two every half-hour. Alternatively, stretch your legs out and move your ankles every few minutes.

Take regular microbreaks, too (see Taking Microbreaks, p.177). This is particularly important if you work at a computer or in a job where you sit or stand in a similar position for long periods.

Balance your heavier and lighter activities. For example, swap vacuuming with dusting, or lawn mowing with light weeding every 15 minutes or so. If you have hand problems, swap repetitive tasks – for example, chopping, cutting, or stirring when cooking, or weeding, pruning, and trowelling when gardening.

This swapping around of tasks will help you to avoid using the same muscle groups in the same repetitive patterns, or continually overworking them for too long. Your joints also get a regular change of position.

Plan your activities more efficiently

Most people have a habitual way of carrying out their regular daily activities. They rarely ask if they can be done more efficiently. If you are in a hurry, you often make more mistakes and waste time – as well as creating more muscle tension and fatigue.

Take the time to plan ahead. For each of the domestic activities you need to do, try out the following task analysis approach (see Task Analysis: Ironing, left):

Q&A

Will planning and pacing my activities mean that I'm just giving in and so make me weaker?

No. Research shows that those who do best in the long term are those who believe they can manage their condition effectively. Look for solutions that help you cope positively and try to avoid getting stuck in frustration. You can genuinely save energy by planning and pacing – then you have more for doing the things you enjoy.

- What steps and different tasks are involved in doing the activity?
- In what order can these steps or tasks be done most efficiently?
- Could you make the activity simpler? Or cut down on the amount that needs to be done?
- Could you do the activity by moving differently or by using differently designed pieces of equipment – for example, one with wheels?
- Would wearing a splint, such as a wrist splint or knee brace, help to reduce the effort required?
- What is the best body position to use when doing the activity?
- Is everything you need easily to hand? If the answer is yes, you will reduce the number of trips around the house or office (or across a room) to collect what you need to do the job.
- Are the items you need stored efficiently? Items regularly used for the same tasks should be stored near one another. Keep items near to the place where they are most frequently used. Arrange your organizers such as drawer dividers, cupboard step shelves, and pull-out shelves so that you can easily reach and pick up items.

Pace your activities

Think of yourself as a battery with a fixed amount of energy for the day. Spend it wisely on what you both need and want to do. Life is about enjoying yourself so it is important for your health to give yourself time for leisure and social activities. Regular rests and breaks act as battery top-ups and regular changes of activity will ease muscle tension.

Balance periods of rest and activity. Take a regular break for a few minutes every 30–45 minutes. If you cannot do this at least take a break for 15 minutes every 2 hours. Sit and let your neck and shoulder muscles relax and let the tension ease away.

Perhaps you think you don't have time to take a rest, or that having a rest means you are giving in to your arthritis. Working for long periods without a break means your body needs a longer recovery time. Research shows that people who take regular short breaks and microbreaks are actually active for longer, more productive, and less tired by the end of the day. Allow yourself to take a break. It's healthier.

Regular rests and breaks act as battery top-ups and regular changes of activity will ease muscle tension.

PRACTICAL TIPS

TAKING MICROBREAKS

Train yourself to take small, regular breaks from whatever you are doing.

- Every 5–10 minutes stretch the joints and muscles you are using for 30–60 seconds.

- Try to move around every 15–30 minutes or so.

- Set up an alarm on your computer, kitchen timer, or mobile phone (or set this to vibrate if you don't want to annoy other people) to remind yourself to take microbreaks. After a few days you will find that the habit of taking breaks starts to form.

WORKING AT A COMPUTER

When you work at a computer, the following advice will help you adopt the best posture so that your joints and muscles do not experience too much stress and strain.

● Buy an ergonomic chair so you can adjust its height. Your knees and the chair must go under the desk to help you sit with your hips at right angles and your back supported.

● Raise the seat or lower the keyboard so you can sit with your shoulders relaxed, elbows comfortably bent, and wrists straight on the keyboard.

● Place the screen at eye level to avoid bending your neck. Voice activation software may help.

● Use an ergonomic keyboard and mouse. If you need to write, clear the desk space rather than leaning awkwardly to one side.

● Don't rest your wrists on the desk edge – use a wrist rest.

● Take microbreaks every 5–10 minutes. Stretch muscles and relax your shoulders and neck.

● Don't clutter your desk area.

● Regular phone users could buy a hands-free phone or headset to avoid leaning to one side.

REDUCE THE STRAIN
Setting up your computer, desk, and chair so that your body is comfortable and not awkward reduces the strain on your joints.

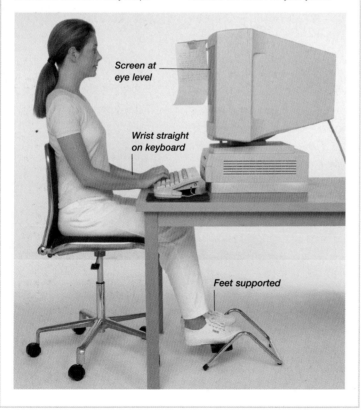

Screen at eye level

Wrist straight on keyboard

Feet supported

Posture

Proper body alignment uses less energy because your weight is balanced centrally. The three curves to the spine – a slight forward curve at the neck, a backward curve at the mid-back, and a forward curve in the lumbar region – help to absorb shocks when you move.

Poor posture increases muscle tension and pain in your neck, shoulder, and lower back. There are two common problems: sitting or standing with your head poked forwards, shoulders hunched, and the lower back slumped; and standing with your knees locked, which arches the lower back and pokes the head forwards.

Standing posture

When you stand, keep your ears in line with your shoulders, which should be relaxed and in line with your hips. Keep your hips in line with your knees and ankles, with your knees very slightly relaxed (not locked rigid) and your weight evenly distributed over your feet.

Sitting posture

When you sit, keep your head upright with your ears over your relaxed shoulders. Relax your upper back, too, and keep it over your hips. Make sure your hips and knees are at right angles (check your seat is not too low). Evenly distribute your weight

Keep your back as straight as you can.

Bend your knees.

Squat down on your haunches.

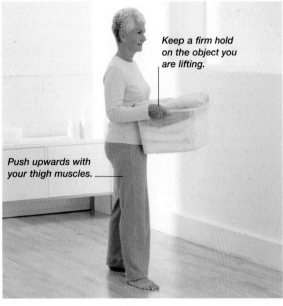

Keep a firm hold on the object you are lifting.

Push upwards with your thigh muscles.

GETTING INTO POSITION
If you have to lift a heavy object, first make sure that you get close to it – then squat down on your haunches and bend your knees rather than your back.

LIFTING THE OBJECT
Check you have a firm hold on the object. Tighten your stomach muscles. Keep the weight close to your body and push upwards using your thigh muscles rather than your back muscles.

across your bottom (not leaning to one side), and ensure your bottom is to the back of the chair seat so your back is supported. Finally, put your feet flat on the floor.

You spend considerable time sitting down so make sure your chairs and sofa are good quality. Poor quality furniture and a slumped posture put extra strain on your joints and back (see right).

Moving and lifting

Avoid moving and lifting heavy objects whenever possible, particularly if you have knee and hip problems. There are safe ways to lift heavy items (see above). If you have to lift objects as part of

your job your employer must by law provide you with training and equipment to make this easier.

Walking

Invest in a pair of good shoes for walking (see p.70). These should have shock-absorbing soles or insoles, a continuous sole with a slightly bevelled heel, and firm support over the top of the foot (either laces or straps).

Many people with foot and leg problems habitually look down at the ground in front of their feet when walking, as they are worried about tripping up. Train yourself to look ahead a few yards to help with your posture.

PRACTICAL TIPS

SEATING CHECKPOINTS

● Your chair or sofa should have a firm seat. Put a board under a saggy sofa seat and change the seat cushion for firmer foam.

● The height of your seat should allow you to sit so that your hips and knees are at right angles.

● Make sure that you have a supportive back rest – preferably up to shoulder and head height so you can relax your head and neck. Check that you have good back support, too – use a small cushion for your lower back if this helps.

Children and special risk groups

For a long time, many people thought arthritis was a condition that primarily affected elderly people. This perception is gradually changing as it becomes clear that arthritis affects other parts of the population in significant numbers.

Arthritis in children can be hard to detect but often develops in a similar way to arthritis in adults. What is different is that children have special needs that must be addressed if they are to grow up as normally as possible.

Foremost among the groups at special risk are post-menopausal women, who seem to be prone to arthritis and osteoporosis. Managing the menopause with hormone replacements can help, but it brings risks of its own.

Obesity and excessive physical activity that puts joints under repeated strain increase the risk of osteoarthritis – a risk that is reduced by losing weight and stopping the repeated activity. People who inherit a predisposition to arthritis can expect to benefit from improved medication and advances in surgical treatments.

Arthritis in children

Few people realize that arthritis affects children as well as adults. In fact, juvenile arthritis seems to catch everyone by surprise, probably because it is easy to overlook and difficult to diagnose. It may take months or years to confirm a diagnosis of arthritis in a child, let alone start effective treatment. However, children with arthritis can benefit from all kinds of therapeutic care and support, while at the same time receiving help for their special needs – at school, home, and at play.

If your child experiences pain in one or more joints he or she may not necessarily have arthritis.

Types of childhood arthritis

Each year, arthritis will affect approximately one child in every thousand – about 12,000 children in the UK. Most of these cases are generally mild and self-limiting, which means they do not get worse over time. More severe types of arthritis affect approximately one child in every 10,000.

Juvenile arthritis is the classic example of inflammatory arthritis in children. However, reactive arthritis, septic arthritis, and some other forms of adult arthritis (see pp.14–25) can also affect children.

Juvenile arthritis

Most of the arthritis in children is due to this group of inflammatory disorders. Also known as juvenile idiopathic arthritis or juvenile rheumatoid arthritis, it involves pain, inflammation, and swelling in at least one joint. Juvenile arthritis may run in families and seems to result from an abnormal response of the immune system.

Depending on the joints involved in the early months of disease and the involvement of other organs, juvenile arthritis is divided into five main types:

■ **OLIGOARTHRITIS** At the start of this condition, fewer than four joints are involved. For example, a young child (perhaps 2 or 3 years of age) may have a swollen knee or ankle, which appears without injury or explanation. This type accounts for about half of the cases of juvenile arthritis.

Often, the arthritis is mild but it may be associated with uveitis. This eye condition, in which the eyes become inflamed, is not necessarily painful, but may result in scarring and damage to the child's eyesight if left untreated.

■ **POLYARTHRITIS** At least 5 joints are involved from the start in this type, which can begin in children of any age, even babies a few months old. Some but not all children with polyarthritis test positive for rheumatoid factor (see p.41).

■ **SYSTEMIC ARTHRITIS** This type accounts for 10–20 per cent of cases. The condition often starts with a rash and a high fever, which varies throughout the day and is

often absent for many hours. In some children, the condition vanishes without returning, while in others the fevers and rash clear up, but the arthritis progresses over time and can become severe. It may involve the internal organs and, rarely, can be life threatening.

■ **ENTHESITIS-RELATED ARTHRITIS** This type involves the spine, hips, and the entheses (the points where tendons attach to bones). It mainly affects boys over 8 years of age.

■ **PSORIATIC ARTHRITIS** This type involves children who have both arthritis and psoriasis (see p.22).

Other causes of joint pain

If your child experiences pain in one or more joints he or she may not necessarily have arthritis. The pain might be due to a condition that affects the mechanical way the joint works or to a chronic pain syndrome of unknown cause, such as fibromyalgia (see p.27).

Several different diseases can cause mechanical problems. Some are rare inherited disorders that involve either the protein collagen or another part of the connective tissue. Others are blood problems, such as sickle cell disease, or minor musculoskeletal complaints, such as Osgood-Schlatter disease, which causes inflammation and pain in front of the shinbone (tibia) below the knee.

Occasionally, children with leukaemia develop features that are very similar to the onset of

Juvenile arthritis sometimes runs in families and seems to result from an abnormal response of the body's immune system.

Q&A

Can a child who has juvenile arthritis develop osteoporosis later in life?

Yes. Children who have been badly affected by juvenile arthritis can later develop osteoporosis (see p.35). If doctors are concerned they may use scans called DEXA (dual energy X-ray absorptiometry) to identify it early. Treatment for the osteoporosis may involve bisphosphonate drugs and calcium, and vitamin D supplements may also be prescribed.

childhood arthritis. An arthritic kind of joint pain may be a feature of inflammatory bowel disease, such as Crohn's disease.

Rheumatic fever may cause a type of arthritis involving several, or even many, joints. However, this is rare and occurs in fewer than 1 in 100,000 children in industrialized countries.

BLOOD TESTS

In general, blood tests for children who may or may not have arthritis are the same tests as those for an adult. They analyse the cell content of the blood – red blood cells, white blood cells, and platelets – and measure the erythrocyte sedimentation rate (ESR) and the levels of auto-antibodies, such as rheumatoid factor, and antinuclear antibodies (see p.41).

BLOOD TEST	REASON FOR TEST
Blood count	To measure the level of haemoglobin – low levels may indicate anaemia, a blood disorder that might have a link to arthritis. High levels of white blood cells and blood platelets may indicate infection or inflammation.
Liver function	To measure the level of some enzymes to check the liver is working properly and to see if it can deal with drugs such as methotrexate.
Kidney function	To measure the level of waste products and salts to check the kidneys are working properly.
Erythrocyte sedimentation rate test (see p.41)	To assess the body's response to a damaging situation, such as inflammation or infection.
Auto-antibodies	To look for auto-antibodies, such as rheumatoid factor and antinuclear antibodies. These may be able to help diagnose the different types of juvenile idiopathic arthritis.
C-reactive protein test (CRP)	To measure the level of C-reactive protein, which is a protein produced by the liver when there is acute inflammation.

Signs to look out for

Arthritis may be hard to diagnose in a child and the first features can be very non-specific. For example, they may be generally unwell or complain of pain.

Arthritis changes the way a child walks or uses his or her arms, legs, hands, and feet. Pain often limits the movement of an affected joint, although younger children will not always complain of pain. If the legs are involved the child may start to limp or walk with difficulty.

Another sign you can look out for is swelling in a child's joint, especially if it is accompanied by pain and stiffness. Such stiffness is particularly concerning when it persists, or is worse in the morning or after a sleep.

Diagnosis

If your doctor suspects that your child has arthritis, he or she will arrange for some blood tests (see left) and some body scans to help confirm a diagnosis.

Blood tests

Just as with adults, a positive result for any blood test does not necessarily confirm that your child has arthritis. Many children with juvenile arthritis have neither rheumatoid factor nor antinuclear antibodies in their blood. It is also true that many children with conditions other than arthritis can

IMAGES OF JOINTS
X-rays, MRI scans, and ultrasound images can help doctors to look closely at joints to see if they are damaged or swollen.

have either rheumatoid factor or antinuclear antibodies (see p.41).

Nevertheless, the presence of either antinuclear antibodies or rheumatoid factor is highly suggestive of juvenile arthritis. A quarter of children with arthritis, particularly oligoarthritis, test positive for antinuclear antibodies. Rheumatoid factor usually indicates polyarthritis that will continue into adult life.

Children with systemic arthritis invariably have a high ESR reading (see p.41). It is usually high in polyarthritis, too, but often normal in children with oligoarthritis.

Taking images

To help confirm a diagnosis or assess the severity of arthritis, your child may need an X–ray or to have a magnetic resonance imaging (MRI) or ultrasound scan, which can show the extent of joint inflammation. They can identify the presence of an inflamed synovium in one or more joints or show the presence of excessive fluid within a joint.

Managing a child's arthritis

In some hospitals a child with arthritis will be looked after by a dedicated paediatric rheumatologist (who is a paediatrician specially trained in managing arthritis). In other hospitals, the role is shared between a dedicated adult rheumatologist with special interest in children and a general paediatrician. These highly qualified consultants are supported by physiotherapists (see p.46) and occupational therapists (see p.144).

Arthritis may be hard to diagnose in a child and the first features can be very non-specific.

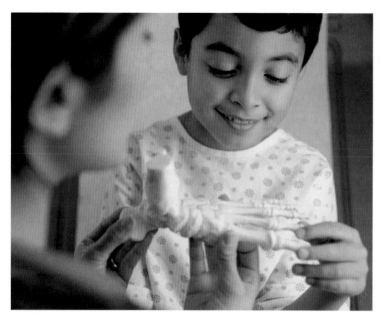

TALKING ABOUT JOINTS
Children with arthritis can enjoy finding out how their joints work, especially if their doctor takes the time to tell them.

The main goals of this care team are to manage your child's arthritis while simultaneously keeping the child in good physical condition and an active part of your family and community. To help the team achieve these goals, your child is treated to reduce swelling and pain, maintain the movement in affected joints, and prevent complications before they arise or resolve them when they do.

Non-steroidal anti-inflammatory drugs

Many suitable non-steroidal anti-inflammatory drugs (NSAIDs), such as ibuprofen, diclofenac, and naproxen, can be prescribed by your child's doctor. Children are not usually treated with aspirin because it may cause bleeding problems, stomach upset, liver problems, or Reye's syndrome.

NSAIDs are effective in reducing pain and stiffness, but do not have any long-term impact on the disease. They also cause multiple side-effects, particularly stomach problems and ulcers.

Disease-modifying anti-rheumatic drugs

When NSAIDs no longer relieve symptoms, disease-modifying anti-rheumatic drugs (DMARDs) may be prescribed. These can relieve symptoms and slow the progress of juvenile idiopathic arthritis when it becomes a long-term illness. They take weeks or months to have an effect, so are usually given together with an NSAID.

The same DMARDs are used in children as are used in adults (see p.83). Methotrexate is preferred by rheumatologists because the small doses needed to relieve symptoms rarely bring on its potentially dangerous side-effects. The most serious complication is liver damage, which can be avoided by regular blood screening tests and careful follow-up. Occasionally, if a child develops a chest problem, such as a persistent dry cough, the methotrexate is discontinued.

Steroids

When a child's arthritis is severe and uncontrolled, or when the inflammation affects internal organs, rheumatologists may add steroids such as prednisolone to existing treatments. Steroids can

Q&A

"Do children who are treated with steroids grow up to be shorter than normal adults?"

This is usually true. In one study, nearly half of adults with previous systemic juvenile idiopathic arthritis who were treated with steroids for at least 2 years during childhood had a final height that was substantially below their projected target height. More than 80 per cent of the adults were shorter than anticipated.

be given by mouth or by injections into a vein (intravenously) or into the muscles (intramuscularly).

Steroids are very effective in the short term, but their effectiveness decreases over time. They have many potential side-effects – for example, they interfere with normal growth, produce a red and round face, cause thinning of the bones (osteoporosis), and increase susceptibility to infections.

Once steroids have started to control severe arthritis symptoms, the dose is gradually reduced and then stopped. Stopping steroids suddenly can be dangerous, so it is important to follow the dosing instructions very carefully.

Biologic agents

Children with severe polyarticular arthritis who have gained little relief from other drugs may be prescribed a biologic agent, such as etanercept and infliximab (see p.86). Rheumatologists usually combine biologic agents with DMARDs such as methotrexate, which rapidly improve symptoms and reduce inflammation.

However, these drugs lower the body's immune response and so increase the risks of infection, such as tuberculosis. The risks, high cost, and potentially serious adverse reactions, mean biologic agents are prescribed with caution.

Physical therapy

A key component of treating a child with arthritis is physical exercise supervised by a physiotherapist. Physical therapy helps to maintain muscle tone and to preserve and recover movement of the joints. When the arthritis is severe, an occupational therapist may recommend the child wears splints (see p.138) to help to maintain growth and reduce pain.

Steroids are very effective in the short term, but their effectiveness decreases over time.

SEEING A PHYSIOTHERAPIST
The expertise of a physiotherapist can help children with arthritis improve muscle tone and maintain mobility in their joints.

AT SCHOOL
Schoolteachers can help children with arthritis conserve energy so that they can concentrate their attention on their education.

Special needs at school

Going to school is an essential part of every child's life and children with arthritis are no exception. It is important, therefore, that their parents, the clinicians involved in their care, and the teachers who educate them work closely together to make sure they receive the best possible education.

It is generally accepted that children with arthritis should remain within the normal school system. However, if your child's arthritis is severe and leads to a stay in hospital for any length of time, provision needs to be made so his or her education can continue during the admission.

Food and diet

Children with arthritis benefit from a good healthy diet (see p.50) with plenty of calories, calcium, and omega-3 fatty acids. They do not need a special diet or any extra vitamins or supplements, although these will do no harm so long as they are taken in moderation.

Complementary therapies

Children with arthritis should always be treated with conventional medicine. Some complementary approaches to health (see pp.108–111) may help a child cope with the stress of living with a chronic illness. However, they are not strongly supported by research evidence. Always ask your doctor for reassurance. If he or she considers a particular approach has value and will not cause harm, you can incorporate it into your child's treatment plan.

Moving around

At school, your child may need special consideration because of difficulties with writing (see p.189) or moving around as quickly as other children. Your child may need help to conserve as much energy as possible for schoolwork. Transport to and from school is important, too, all the more so in the morning when joint stiffness can be acute. Going to school often means carrying around heavy bags, so ask for an extra locker or if your child can keep textbooks at home.

When your child is at school, moving quickly between classes can be difficult. Ask the teachers if they will let your child leave lessons a few minutes before other pupils. It may be impossible for schools to organize, but the ideal situation would be for children with arthritis to attend lessons on the ground floor in a reasonably small area that keeps walking distances short and avoids stairs.

Gaining confidence

Break times and PE lessons can be a challenge. Some active playtime and indoor activities with friends are essential to avoid feelings of isolation and to reduce stiffness.

However, children with active arthritis may be unable to exercise much and they often feel uncertain or embarrassed about their illness. Encourage your child to talk about his or her worries with a friend or a sympathetic teacher and so gain more confidence about joining in.

Special needs at play

Arthritis does not have to prevent a child from participating in active play, which is an essential part of growing up and remains vital for health and growth. While every child needs a daily dose of active play, the physical benefits are invaluable for children with stiff and sore joints. Active play helps maintain energy and increases joint flexibility as well as muscle strength. You cannot reasonably expect a young child to take part in repetitive exercises, but you can usually get him or her to play.

With some creativity and a little ingenuity, it is possible to persuade every child with arthritis to be actively engaged in play. Your child needs to be careful with exercise choices. For instance, it is best to

PRACTICAL TIPS

SPECIAL WRITING NEEDS

Arthritis in the hands and wrists can make writing hard, slow, or painful. The following tips may help a child with schoolwork:

- Allow a child to take breaks from writing.

- A splint will support the child's wrist and encourage the best position for writing, taking the strain off the joints and letting the fingers and thumb move more freely.

- Encourage keyboard skills so a child can use a computer (with a wrist support) instead of writing.

- Provide special grips that can be fitted to pens, pencils, etc.

THE IMPORTANCE OF PLAY
Active play that avoids overuse of particularly hot or inflamed joints is essential to the health and growth of every child with arthritis.

Joining a support group can provide the family with help, advice, and guidance as well as the chance to talk to other young people and parents of children with arthritis.

TALK TO YOUR CHILD
Spending time talking to a child with arthritis will help him or her understand the nature of the illness and will bring you closer together as a family.

avoid contact sports and activities that will overuse one part of the body. It is also important to avoid activities that stress those joints that are hot or inflamed. However, it is also essential to encourage activities that keep children with their friends.

Special needs at home

Without question, arthritis in children imposes physical and psychological stresses on family life. Even the most stable of families struggle to establish and maintain a sensible balance in the order of things. When the child needs special care, the strain on keeping that balance is increased exponentially. Family relationships may suffer when parents set aside too much time for the child.

When the arthritis is particularly bad, the child feels too unwell to take part in any activity, causing complex problems within the family. Try to make adjustments and contingency plans. The family needs to accept such uncertainties with equanimity, and to encourage ideas for activities on active days and quiet days.

Family members should try to help by treating the child with arthritis as normally as possible, whilst ensuring that he or she receives suitable medical care. Vitally important, too, is the need to explain to the child that getting arthritis is no-one's fault. Occasionally, children believe that their arthritis is a repayment for something they did.

Joining a support group can provide the family with help, advice, and guidance as well as the chance to talk to other young people and parents of children with arthritis.

Long-term outlook

Overall, the prognosis for juvenile arthritis is relatively good. With modern techniques of treatment and management, most children do very well.

The long-term outlook for pauciarticular juvenile arthritis is very good. However, this is not true of polyarthritis because there is a substantial risk of progressive and destructive arthritis as well as joint deformities. This is especially true if rheumatoid factor is present in the blood (see p.41).

The long-term outlook of systemic arthritis depends on the organs affected and if it progresses to polyarticular disease.

Complications can be very worrying in a small number

of children. Complications include infection, inflammation of the heart, and kidney disease.

The effect on growth

Many children with juvenile chronic arthritis, especially those with systemic or polyarthritis, do not grow normally. One typical feature is a small lower jaw and a small chin.

The main causes of affected growth are chronic inflammation and steroid treatment (see p.186), with other contributions from poor nutrition that comes with decreased appetite as well as limited physical activity. However, active treatment and the careful use of minimal doses of steroids can help to reduce the degree of retarded growth.

The longer juvenile arthritis continues, the more likely the inflamed joints and surrounding muscles and tendons will become damaged. What effect prolonged inflammation has depends on which joints are most involved.

Typical problems include the inability to bend and straighten the knees properly, shortened legs, and damage to the small joints of the hand. Sometimes, the joints in the neck are damaged.

However, orthopaedic surgeons have developed techniques that can replace a joint that fails (see p.92), release a joint that cannot straighten properly, and remove excessive cartilage from a joint.

Serious complications

Some children with arthritis can develop serious organ problems, due either to the disease or its treatment with drugs. Problems include an inflamed pericardium (the membrane around the heart) and kidney failure. Inflammation of the blood vessels (see p.34) can affect many different organs.

Uveitis, in which the uvea layer of the eye becomes inflamed, is potentially debilitating and can result in blindness. Expert care and monitoring from eye surgeons can minimize the risks.

Children who have prolonged and widespread inflammation that is left untreated can accumulate a protein called amyloid throughout the body. This causes failure of individual organs, such as the kidneys. However, with modern treatments this complication is becoming increasingly rare.

ENCOURAGING GROWTH
Physical activity, along with good nutrition and careful use of steroids, can encourage growth and minimize the chances of retarded growth.

People at special risk

Some people are more prone than others to developing one of the many forms of arthritis. Women represent the largest group because they are destined to experience the menopause, a time of hormonal change that makes their metabolism more vulnerable to developing arthritis. Other special risk groups include people who put their joints under persistent or repetitive strain – athletes, manual workers, and obese individuals – and people who are genetically predisposed to arthritis.

HRT not only helps to increase the density of bone but may also prevent osteoarthritis of the knee.

Post-menopause and arthritis

Arthritis affects more women in the general population than men. But age is an important factor in this picture; the biggest proportion of women with arthritis are post-menopausal. This is the time in a woman's life when she is most likely to suffer from osteoarthritis or rheumatoid arthritis. As if this susceptibility was not enough, a post-menopausal woman is at an increased risk of developing osteoporosis, too.

After the menopause a woman's body changes in many different ways because her ovaries have stopped producing the hormones oestrogen and progesterone. Among the many effects that this hormonal change appears to have is an increased risk of developing osteoarthritis, particularly of the knees and hands. As a result, osteoarthritis is much more common in women of this age (late 40s to early 50s) than men.

The link between oestrogen and osteoarthritis is still not completely understood, but many studies seem to suggest that one does exist. Australian researchers, for example, have found that hormone replacement therapy (HRT) not

Q&A

If I take corticosteroids what are the risks that I will go on to develop osteoporosis?

Anyone who takes corticosteroids for more than 3 months has an increased risk of developing osteoporosis, and the risk increases if you:

● Have a family history of the disease.

● Have had previous fractures.

● Have ever had anorexia nervosa.

● Smoke or abuse alcohol.

● Take certain medications, such as the blood thinner heparin.

only helps to increase the density of bone but may also prevent osteoarthritis of the knee.

Doctors in the US found that when women are receiving treatments for conditions that deplete the oestrogen in the body, as with some breast cancer drugs, they are more prone to developing osteoarthritis. However, the possible risks associated with taking HRT (see p.195) mean that it is unlikely to be recommended by doctors as a treatment for osteoarthritis alone.

Osteoporosis

Osteoporosis, which literally means "porous bone", is a disease that causes the bones in the body to become less dense and more fragile (see p.35). In women, the hormone oestrogen plays an important role in helping to keep

bones strong and so the loss of oestrogen after the menopause significantly increases loss of bone density and consequently the risk of osteoporosis.

One in three women over the age of 50 will develop osteoporosis. Women who have had an early menopause, a hysterectomy (removal of the uterus), or their ovaries removed before they reach the menopause are also at risk of developing osteoporosis.

Rheumatoid arthritis and osteoporosis

Women are two to three times more likely to develop rheumatoid arthritis than men. At the same time, if you have rheumatoid arthritis you are also more likely to develop osteoporosis.

There may be several reasons for this link. First, the inflammation

HEALTHY BONE
Normal spongy bone (left) contains trabeculae, which are like struts that are both light and strong. Bone marrow fills the space in between the trabeculae.

OSTEOPOROSIS
In osteoporosis (left), the fabric of the spongy bone tissue becomes less dense and more brittle. Here, a vertebra is affected with osteoporosis, made visible by many small dark areas of bone.

and pain of rheumatoid arthritis may prevent or deter women from regular exercise, which can also have a negative effect on the strength of their bones.

Second, studies show that rheumatoid arthritis can make you more susceptible to osteoporosis because of the bone loss that may

occur around affected joints. Finally, if you take corticosteroids for the pain and inflammation in rheumatoid arthritis there is a significant risk that you will have some reduction in bone density.

Preventing osteoporosis

The best way of preventing osteoporosis, or at least slowing its progress, is to take enough calcium and vitamins, especially vitamin D, and to do plenty of regular weight-bearing exercise. Your doctor may prescribe drugs called bisphosphonates, which are bone-protecting agents.

Calcium

This mineral is vital for the health of your bones. Good sources of calcium (see left) include foods such as dairy products. You don't need full-fat versions because low-fat dairy products contain as much and sometimes even more calcium as their fattier counterparts.

You also find calcium in Brazil nuts, dried beans, dark-green leafy vegetables, such as spinach, kale and broccoli, as well as in tinned salmon and sardines that contain the bones. Some foods such as bread and orange juice are fortified with extra calcium.

If you don't think you can include enough calcium in your diet, add a little powdered milk to some recipes, such as puddings or soups, or ask your doctor about taking a supplement.

SOURCES OF CALCIUM

The average recommended daily amount (RDA) by the government is currently 700mg of calcium for men and women, but if you already have osteoporosis you may need up to 1,200mg. The chart below provides some guidelines on how much calcium is present in certain foods.

FOOD	WEIGHT/VOLUME	CALCIUM CONTENT
Full-fat milk	190ml (1/3 pint)	224 mg
Semi-skimmed milk	190ml (1/3 pint)	231 mg
Skimmed milk	190ml (1/3 pint)	235 mg
Low-fat yoghurt	150g (5oz)	225 mg
Ice cream	112g (4oz)	134 mg
Cheddar cheese	28g (1oz)	202 mg
Boiled spinach	112g (4oz)	179 mg
Baked beans	112g (4oz)	59 mg
White bread (1 slice)	28g (1oz)	33 mg
1 large orange		58 mg
Dried apricots	100g (3 1/2 oz)	92 mg
Brazil nuts	100g (3 1/2 oz)	170 mg
Whitebait (fried)	56g (2 oz)	482 mg
Salmon (tinned)	56g (2 oz)	52 mg

GET SOME SUN
Regular sunlight helps you to produce vitamin D, which in turn helps you absorb calcium.

Vitamin D

This vitamin plays an important part in helping your body to absorb calcium. If you spend time outside in the sunlight on a regular basis you will be able to make all the vitamin D you need.

Dietary sources of vitamin D include egg yolks, some vitamin-enriched foods, and supplements. There is some limited evidence that vitamin D may be helpful in osteoarthritis, too.

Exercise

Regular exercise builds up the strength of your bones and muscles. Weight-bearing exercise is the best kind because it forces you to work against gravity and helps to minimize the loss of minerals, such as calcium, from the bones. Walking, climbing stairs, and dancing are all good examples of beneficial weight-bearing exercise.

However, if you already have developed osteoporosis, walking for half an hour a day is best because it puts the least stress on your bones. Taking exercise can be off-putting if you have arthritis, but it is vital that joints are given enough movement to prevent further damage and pain (see pp.64–73 and pp.158–171).

Hormone replacement therapy

Hormone replacement therapy, or HRT, is the artificial replacement of the hormones oestrogen and progesterone that are lost during and after the menopause.

Many women, regardless of whether or not they already have arthritis, experience a range of bothersome or unpleasant symptoms both before and after the menopause. These symptoms include hot flushes, dry skin, irritability, and even depression.

REGULAR EXERCISE
Taking exercise regularly is a crucial part of maintaining the health of your bones and preventing osteoporosis.

HRT PATCH
Adhesive patches are a simple and effective way of delivering HRT drugs slowly and directly into the bloodstream.

HRT is not recommended as a drug therapy for the treatment of osteoporosis or heart disease alone.

Some women also experience a loss of sex drive and discomfort during sex.

HRT is the standard treatment for these symptoms. It is taken in the form of tablets, patches worn against the skin, or implants placed just under the skin.

Women who have undergone the menopause early, or have had a hysterectomy or their ovaries removed, are also offered HRT. Most women will take oestrogen with progesterone, although oestrogen-only and progesterone-only versions are available.

HRT has been shown to protect against osteoporosis. It is also possible that it may offer some protection against osteoarthritis in post-menopausal women.

The risks of HRT

Taking HRT has been associated with several serious health risks, including breast cancer, blood clots, and cardiovascular disease.

■ **BREAST CANCER** If HRT is taken for less than 5 years there doesn't appear to be any increased risk of breast cancer, but after this time there is a small increase. A major study, known as the Million Women Study, appeared to show the biggest risk of breast cancer is posed by HRT when it combines oestrogen and progesterone.

When a woman has not had a hysterectomy, progesterone protects against endometrial cancer, so doctors will still advise her to take the combined hormones. Taking HRT does not seem to increase the risk of breast cancer when women take it at a younger age than the norm – for example, after an early hysterectomy or a premature menopause. The 5-year risk period seems to begin from the age of 50. After 5 years, for all women, the risk appears to be the same as for someone who is not taking HRT.

■ **BLOOD CLOTS** Taking HRT appears to carry a slightly higher than normal risk of developing a blood clot, or venous thromboembolism (VTE). If you are already in a risk group for VTE, you should fully discuss with your doctor whether HRT is suitable for you. There is some evidence that, in these cases, the non-oral forms, such as patches, carry a lower risk.

■ **CARDIOVASCULAR DISEASE** The received wisdom on taking HRT has been that it protects women from both heart disease and strokes. However, studies have suggested this benefit is less clear cut, and many experts now believe HRT provides no protection. There is some evidence that, in the long term, the risks of taking HRT may outweigh its benefits, although this remains controversial.

Is HRT worth the risk?
In the UK the consensus seems to be that for women who experience the more distressing symptoms of the menopause or early menopause, the benefits of taking HRT usually outweigh the risks.

HRT is not recommended as a drug therapy for the treatment of osteoporosis or heart disease alone. With any form of medication, it is important that you talk to your doctor about your particular circumstances and whether the drug in question is right for you.

Sporting risks

Super-fit people, such as athletes, footballers, and basketball players, who constantly train and play sport regularly, have an increased risk of arthritis. This is because any trauma on a joint – whether from persistent repetitive movement, overuse, or a sports injury – can make the joint more susceptible to developing arthritis.

Depending on which joint is overused, the severity of the trauma, and the intensity of the inflammation that is produced as

PLAYING FOOTBALL
The sudden twists, turns, and tackles in a game of football can expose players to joint damage that could lead to arthritis later.

PRACTICAL TIPS

AVOIDING INJURIES
● Play the sport or practise the exercise that suits you. If taking part in an activity makes you uncomfortable you may increase the risk of getting injured.

● Buy the appropriate gear and equipment for your chosen sport or activity and you will feel much more comfortable. Don't struggle to get by with worn-out or second-rate footwear, clothes, and equipment.

● Always warm up before you start and cool down afterwards.

● Try to build up the muscles around your joints.

● Avoid repetitive activities and try to exercise different muscles and joints.

● Don't ignore the little stresses and strains in your body. If you feel a pain, stop what you're doing.

● If you do sustain an injury, don't just ignore it and think it will be alright in the morning. Consult a doctor and get it looked at so that it can heal properly.

a result of the damage to cartilage and soft tissues, a degree of osteoarthritis is likely.

Repetitive trauma carries a high risk of future problems. One example is osteoarthritis of the knee (see p.17) that develops in former professional footballers, many of whom may have had replacement knee surgery (see p.94) at a relatively early age.

Occupational risks

Occupations in which there is repetitive knee bending or an increased risk of injury to the knee joints, particularly a repetitive injury, are associated with the development of osteoarthritis later in life. Examples include heavy manual work in such industries as forestry, construction, and agriculture.

Other joints that may be affected by overuse and repetitive injuries include hips, wrists, shoulders, and lower back (see pp.28–31). Dancers and musicians are particularly prone to overuse of their joints – for example, the bowing shoulder of violinists and the hands of pianists are commonly affected.

MECHANICAL VIBRATION
Drills, jack hammers, and other sources of mechanical vibration can cause carpal tunnel syndrome and repetitive strain injury.

Obesity

People who are obese are at much greater risk of developing knee osteoarthritis than people who are a healthy weight for their height. This is especially so for women. Obesity is usually defined as having a body mass index (BMI) of 30 or more. You can calculate your BMI by measuring your height in metres and weight in kilograms (see opposite). Studies have shown that for every increase in BMI above 27, the risk of developing knee osteoarthritis increases by 15 per cent. Losing weight may help reduce this risk (see p.62).

Being overweight or obese can lead to osteoarthritis in several ways. First, being overweight increases the amount of force on weight-bearing joints, such as the knees. Second, the fatty tissues may alter the person's balance of hormones, which could affect cartilage and bone tissues. Third, obese people have relatively weak muscles, are less fit than normal, and injure themselves more often.

Ethnic groups

The relationship between ethnicity and arthritis is complex. From a genetic point of view, a particular ethnic group may be predisposed or more prone to a particular type of arthritis. Added to this is the fact that different groups receive – for

CALCULATING BODY MASS INDEX (BMI)

Body mass index (BMI) is the relationship of your weight in kilograms divided by the square of your height in metres. For example, a man who weighs 100kg and is 1.8m tall has a BMI of 30.86. A woman who weighs 70kg and is 1.6m tall has a BMI of 27.34. The chart below will help to place your BMI in one of four groups, from underweight to obese.

whatever reason – different levels of medical care, which affects the way their arthritis is treated.

Finally, members of different ethnic groups respond in different ways to apparently similar clinical problems. For example, the way individuals respond to pain and disability is very dependent on their overall view of the world and the support they receive from their family and community.

Ethnicity and rheumatoid arthritis

Variations in the frequency of rheumatoid arthritis have been studied in detail in different ethnic groups. In most Western countries, the disease affects an average of about 1 per cent of adults (1.5 per cent of women and 0.6 per cent of men). Lower rates of rheumatoid arthritis have been reported in China, Japan, parts of Greece, and rural Africa. It seems particularly uncommon in West Africa.

Conversely, there appears to be a high prevalence in several Native American populations, such as the Tlingit of Southeast Alaska, the Yakima of Central Washington, and the Pima of Arizona. The high rate of rheumatoid arthritis in these populations leads to speculation about their unique

From a genetic point of view, a particular ethnic group may be predisposed or more prone to a particular type of arthritis.

genetic or environmental factors. The clinical features of rheumatoid arthritis in these Native Americans are different from those of the normal population: the disease is more severe, often starts at a younger age and a family history is more common. This prevalence and severity strongly suggests that genetics play an important role.

Ethnicity and osteoarthritis

Some forms of osteoarthritis, such as generalized osteoarthritis that involves the hand, are found predominantly in Caucasians. Conversely, good evidence indicates that hand and foot osteoarthritis is uncommon in Africans. However, the situation is complex, as knee osteoarthritis is common in African Americans. Finally, some groups have very low rates of osteoarthritis of the hip, including Chinese and Japanese populations.

Inherited markers or traits

The inherited nature of arthritis has been known for many years, mainly from family studies that show that if one member of a family has rheumatoid arthritis or ankylosing spondylitis it is more likely to be found in other family members. Studies of twins lend even more support to this inheritance: when one twin has the disease the other is more likely

For many years, rheumatologists have known that genetics play a strong role in ankylosing spondylitis.

to have it if the twins are identical rather than non-identical.

Studying the genetics of people with arthritis suggests that there are marker genes or traits in their chromosomes, especially the HLA–DR4 marker in rheumatoid arthritis and the HLA–B27 marker in ankylosing spondylitis.

HLA–DR4 in rheumatoid arthritis

Genetic studies in rheumatoid arthritis have concentrated mainly on white blood cells and, in particular, a group of genes that is called the major histocompatibility complex (MHC).

Scientists have discovered that one of these genes, known as HLA–DR4, is present in some people with rheumatoid arthritis but not others. They think that there is a link between this discovery and the geographical variation of rheumatoid arthritis.

Q&A

Both my father and my mother suffered from arthritis – does this mean that I will develop it, too?

Not necessarily. According to research, some forms of arthritis may well be linked to certain genes and may therefore be inherited. But this is not inevitable. There do seem to be other triggers such as infections that can bring on arthritis. Besides, rheumatologists are uncertain about the causes of many types of arthritis.

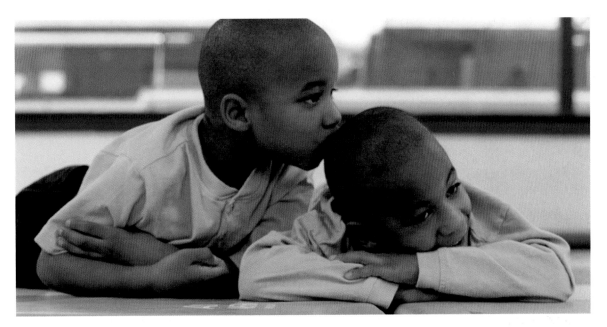

Evidence suggests that people who have the HLA–DR4 gene have rheumatoid arthritis more severely and are more likely to have rheumatoid nodules and erosion of the bones within their joints.

As the gene is important in determining how the immune system works, scientists thought they were on the verge of a breakthrough. To date, they have been unable to unravel the story further. As a result, the knowledge that someone has the HLA-DR4 gene has not yet influenced the treatment of rheumatoid arthritis.

HLA–B27 in ankylosing spondylitis

For many years, rheumatologists have known that genetics play a strong role in ankylosing spondylitis. In the early 1970s, scientists showed that this was due to the presence of a gene known as HLA–B27, which also belongs to the MHC group.

About 95 per cent of people with ankylosing spondylitis have this genetic marker, compared to 8 per cent of the general population. HLA–B27 is also found, but with less frequency, in other conditions that are associated with ankylosing spondylitis. These include uveitis (eye inflammation) and psoriatic arthritis (see p.22).

One or more environmental triggers lead to ankylosing spondylitis in a minority (about 5–10 per cent) of people who have the HLA–B27 gene. Many of these triggers are likely to be infections, particularly infections in the bowel or pelvis. Those populations with a high rate of rheumatoid arthritis, such as the Pima of Arizona, often have HLA-B27, too.

IDENTICAL TWINS
The genes of identical twins reveal that when one twin develops arthritis the other is more likely to develop it, too.

Long-term outlook

The management and treatment of arthritis has improved greatly over the years, but there has been no cure. This gradual progress is probably the most realistic scenario for the future, too – rather than expecting breakthroughs that lead to a cure, it seems more rational to think in terms of continuing small improvements.

Perhaps the true aim of treating arthritis is to ensure that everyone with arthritis can achieve a good response to treatment while keeping the prospect of disability to a minimum.

Progress in managing arthritis comes with increased prevention, early intervention, and better treatments. In the past, it has also come with a significant increase in the number of arthritis specialists, in the improved access to a range of healthcare professionals, and in the development of many new treatments.

However, most forms of arthritis increase with age – as people continue to live longer they are likely to have more arthritis rather than less. The demographic time bomb underlying the aging of western populations is likely to increase chronic conditions of later life, including arthritis.

The outlook for arthritis

As with many long-term conditions, the outlook for anyone with arthritis is hard to predict. From year to year, changes may affect your prognosis – some for the better, such as new treatment or a spontaneous improvement in symptoms. On the other hand, life with arthritis can get more complicated if new health problems arise or when aging starts to make itself felt. However, one thing is certain. Taking an active part in your own health care will give you the best chance of managing your arthritis well.

Mild osteoarthritis does not necessarily become worse and could remain relatively stable for the rest of your life.

What's likely to happen?

Most people with arthritis have the condition mildly. They can lead full lives, follow careers, sustain relationships, and pursue leisure activities. For the small minority with severe arthritis, life will be more challenging, though there is no reason to limit horizons.

If you are newly diagnosed, you need time to make adjustments both physically and mentally. With the help of healthcare specialists, you can learn more about your condition and find the confidence to cope. What happens in the years after diagnosis depends on the management of your condition, on the type of arthritis you have, and how it affects you as an individual. Although many forms of arthritis have a broad recognizable pattern, no doctor can be certain what your personal prognosis might be.

Osteoarthritis
Mild osteoarthritis (see p.14) does not necessarily get worse and may remain relatively stable for the rest of your life. In later years, your mobility may be about the same as would be normal with aging. You may find your symptoms tend to vary – for example, stiffness and pain may ease in warmer weather.

Rheumatoid arthritis

Most people with rheumatoid arthritis (see p.18) have variable symptoms. The arthritis is active for weeks and months, then dies down or disappears for a while before flaring up again. The amount of damage to the joints depends on the severity of flare-ups and how often they occur.

Eventually, you are likely to have some degree of permanent damage. However, the chances are that you will live relatively normally, and it is important to realize that severe disability is uncommon. Occasionally, flare-ups cease altogether; but if this happens, any joint damage will remain.

Ankylosing spondylitis

The outlook for most people with ankylosing spondylitis (see p.21) is good. Severe disability is not usual, as treatment (especially regular exercise or physiotherapy) is very effective in keeping joint stiffness at bay. If you have the condition, you have a reasonable chance of being only mildly affected in your day-to-day life.

Changes in long-term treatment

You may be taking a drug that suits you and has kept your symptoms well controlled for many years. But sometimes, for reasons not related to arthritis, this drug may stop being an option. From midlife onwards, other health problems start to become more common. In some cases, they are made worse by your arthritis drugs or require medication that interacts with your existing treatment.

For example, if you develop high blood pressure you may not be able to take steroids to reduce inflammation, because they raise blood pressure. Anti-clotting drugs for a cardiovascular disorder cannot be taken with certain types of NSAID, which also have an anti-clotting effect. If you develop a kidney or liver disease, you will not be able to take some disease-modifying anti-rheumatic drugs (see p.83) because their potential side-effects include damage to the kidneys or liver.

If you do need to discontinue an arthritis drug or to take a mixture of drugs for different conditions,

Q&A

Does rheumatoid arthritis put me at greater risk of developing other diseases in the long term?

Possibly. research studies suggest that conditions such as heart disease, osteoporosis, stroke, and infections may be more likely. One reason may be that people with rheumatoid arthritis are not able to exercise freely. In some cases, the drugs for rheumatoid arthritis can raise blood pressure (a risk factor for stroke) or damp down the immune system, making infections more likely.

PRACTICAL TIPS

REDUCING THE RISK OF LONG-TERM PROBLEMS

● Take an active part in managing your arthritis.

● Stay as physically active as possible. Maintain your mobility and exercise your joints and muscles regularly (see pp.158–171).

● Eat a well-balanced diet.

● Keep your weight to a healthy level (see p.199).

● Don't smoke or drink excessively.

● Follow your doctor's instructions and keep taking your medication.

● Make sure you are tested and monitored regularly so that problems can be spotted – and treated – sooner rather than later.

Improved materials and surgical procedures mean that implants now work better for longer than they did in the past.

REGULAR EXERCISE
The importance of regular exercise cannot be emphasized enough – just resist the temptation to overdo it by going beyond reasonable limits.

your doctor will tell you what is best. In some cases, you may need to take drugs for a possibly life-threatening disease at the expense of controlling your arthritis. It is all a question of balance.

Keeping a replacement joint working

Joint replacement surgery can be life-changing, giving back mobility to people who thought they would never enjoy normal activities again. Improved materials and surgical procedures mean that implants now work better for longer than they did in the past. Your implant could serve you well for up to 20 years – but it won't last forever. So what can you expect in the long term?

Inevitably, with wear and tear, replacement joints tend to loosen over time, becoming less efficient or causing pain. If this happens, it may be necessary to perform revision surgery (see p.107) to prevent damage within the joint and possible further disability. Surgery the second time round takes longer and is

more complicated than the initial operation. Recovery is likely to take longer, too.

You can do a lot to get the best from a replacement joint and to protect it from early deterioration. Take regular exercise to keep the implant mobile, but don't be tempted to go beyond reasonable limits, however fit you feel. In particular, avoid high-impact activities or sudden movements that subject the joint to excessive stresses and strains. A fall can seriously damage an implant, so take precautions by making sure your home is safe and free from hazards that are easy to trip over.

Problems in the elderly

Although arthritis is not just a condition that occurs in later life, some forms – particularly osteoarthritis and rheumatoid arthritis – are far more likely to develop in older people. By the time they reach their 50s or 60s, over 30 per cent of people have some symptoms of arthritis.

The frequency of arthritis rises with increasing age: some 60 per cent of those over 85 years old are affected. Because people are living longer – at least, in the developed world – they are more and more often having to deal with the challenges that arise when their arthritis combines with the unique problems of old age.

Reduced movement

The elderly have weaker muscles than younger people, so they find it more difficult to cope with the way arthritis affects their mobility. It is harder for them to stay active enough to maintain strength and fitness through exercise, so their disability is likely to increase. Their movement can be further restricted by joint or bone damage not related to arthritis, such as a fracture of the hip or shoulder caused by a fall. However, in many instances, simple measures such as a programme of supervised walking can make an important difference.

Coping with drug treatment

Drugs for treating arthritis tend to have a more toxic effect in elderly people. This is partly because the older we get the less efficient our bodies become at breaking down drugs. Also, older people are more likely to be taking drugs for other conditions and these may interact with arthritis drugs (see p.205). For this reason, doctors keep the dosages to a minimum and carefully monitor their older patients to watch for reactions.

Living with arthritis

Arthritis won't just go away – but that doesn't mean you have to regard the condition as a life sentence of increasing disability and pain. For one thing, with

ENJOYING PLEASURE
People with arthritis have every reason to enjoy the pleasures of laughter, fun, and happiness.

specialist support available, you have expert help in keeping your symptoms under control. Doctors, therapists, nurses, and researchers work as a team to make your arthritis as manageable as possible.

As one of the most important members of this team you can do a lot to improve your outlook. Even the most highly effective drugs will not work unless you follow your doctor's instructions and take your medication regularly.

Many aspects of general health that make a big difference to your arthritis are under your control, too. For example, you can choose whether or not to exercise to improve strength and mobility, to eat sensibly, to maintain a healthy weight, or to avoid damaging your body by smoking or excess drinking. Good self-management is an essential part of your treatment.

Arthritis in the future

As with many other conditions, scientists are working to find a cure for arthritis. However, no-one expects the discovery of a wonder drug that will cure all symptoms in everyone. But as research progresses, understanding of arthritis in all its diverse forms continues to grow and means the possibility of improvements in the management and treatment of the disease. Ongoing trials are testing powerful new medications and therapies with the potential to significantly reduce the disability caused by arthritis.

Medical scientists are trying to develop appropriate medications in various potential avenues, and are waiting to make significant breakthroughs.

Making progress

Without doubt, considerable progress in treating the various forms of arthritis has been made over the years. Not least, there have been great improvements in three important areas: better surgical techniques to replace joints, an increase in the number of arthritis specialists, and improved access to a range of specialized expertise and healthcare professionals.

Broad lines of research

It is not easy to speculate about the future of arthritis and arthritis care, but there are several broad lines of research. In the simplest approach, clinicians look at ways of maximizing the effectiveness of current treatments, focusing particularly on the timing of drug therapy and how different drugs can be combined.

In another approach, various pharmaceutical companies are working to develop innovative treatments, either by making small improvements to tried and tested drugs or by introducing entirely new ones.

Other avenues of research include studies on the role of genetics in arthritis and the link between infection and joint inflammation.

The development of new drugs

As arthritis is a common and long-lasting disease, and widespread among all populations and age groups, it is a natural target for research into new drugs.

The pharmaceutical industry will continue to research and deliver new drugs and medications to treat the various forms of arthritis. From a commercial point of view, the size of the market means that the financial rewards for success are substantial.

Developing successful new drugs takes pharmaceutical companies many years of painstaking research and is enormously expensive. Most of the drugs they investigate fail to make the grade because their benefits are limited or they have an excessively toxic effect.

However, every decade sees new medications coming to the fore, each with some unique benefits over their predecessors. Not all of these drugs stand the test of time, but most do.

Drug prospects

Trials to test the effectiveness of drugs (see p.213) are valuable because they can focus on the causes of arthritis or of its ultimate effects on joint damage. Medical scientists are trying to develop appropriate medications in various potential avenues, and are waiting to make significant breakthroughs.

■ **ANTIBIOTICS** If medical research revealed that a particular type of arthritis was caused by infection, pharmaceutical companies would try to develop a specific antibiotic to combat it.

■ **DISEASE-MODIFYING DRUGS** A drug that effectively blocks, or inhibits, the enzymes involved in joint damage could have the potential to be a disease-modifying drug in the treatment of osteoarthritis.

■ **ORAL TNF–ALPHA BLOCKERS** Another prospect on the horizon is the development of second generation TNF–alpha blockers (see p.85), which can be taken by mouth. The first generation of these relatively new drugs have to be administered

MEDICAL RESEARCH
Many years of careful medical research are required before a potential drug is fully tested and available for prescription.

MICROSCOPIC EXAMINATION
Medical research, even looking at the effects of a drug on biological tissue through a microscope, is conducted in hygienic conditions.

by injection, although many people with rheumatoid arthritis are happy to accept injections as necessary if their disease is to remain better controlled.

■ **IMPROVED PAINKILLERS** A need that has not yet been met to any great extent is for improved painkillers. There have been many attempts, but almost all have fallen by the wayside for one reason or another. To discover a safe and effective painkiller that causes few side-effects may be impossible.

■ **REVERSING JOINT DAMAGE** The ultimate goal is to design a drug that will reduce or even reverse the joint damage in all types of arthritis. Several potential drugs

have been tried in research studies and, although none has yet proved successful, there is a good chance that the ideal drug will eventually be identified.

Testing biological agents
The most likely area for new drug developments lies in identifying biologic agents (see p.85) that can block, or inhibit, one or more of the pathways in inflammation.

This is a challenging task, as there are a host of different targets in the body, such as the small chemicals called cytokines, that might be relevant. Some 30 or so biological agents are being tested at present, of which at least a quarter, perhaps more, will become available for treating inflammatory arthritis over the next couple of decades.

This research work raises the possibility of discovering more specific biologic agents to target rarer diseases, such as ankylosing spondylitis, psoriatic arthritis, reactive arthritis, and lupus.

Eventually, medical research may even lead to the evolution of a combination therapy (see p.87) in which several biologic agents – each affecting a different cytokine – are used to suppress or even cure rheumatoid arthritis.

Investigating infections

Doctors are learning more about the link between infections and arthritis. In some people, infection causes a fault in the immune system so that substances produced by the body to fight the infection also attack the tissue of healthy joints – and scientists are trying to find out exactly why.

Their experiments have shown that it may be possible to block the damaging effects of a faulty immune system without affecting its protective mechanism.

This avenue of research could have exciting implications, both for identifying people at risk of developing arthritis and for the prevention and treatment of arthritis in the future.

Stem cell transplants

A pioneering procedure causing much interest and excitement is stem cell transplantation. Stem cells are immature cells, formed in bone marrow, with the potential to develop into specialized cells, like those directing the immune system or forming joint cartilage.

One approach uses stem cells to rebuild the immune system. Stem cells are taken from a person's blood, purified, and stored. Then the existing immune system is destroyed by drugs. Subsequently, stem cells are put back into the person's blood. If all goes well, these stem cells form a new healthy immune system.

In rheumatoid arthritis the immune system has become faulty, and stem cell transplantation can

STEM CELLS
Depending on the biochemical signal that it receives, each of the stem cells in this clump has the potential to grow and develop into any type of cell in the body.

have dramatic effects. Symptoms of arthritis may be greatly reduced or even disappear altogether. The treatment has enormous potential.

A second approach uses stem cells to repair specialized tissues such as the cartilage of a joint that has been damaged by a sporting injury or osteoarthritis.

Risks of stem cell transplants

Transplanting stem cells to rebuild the immune system is risky because it leaves the individual temporarily without immunity to minor infections. He or she must remain isolated in hospital until a new immune system is established. It is also possible the stem cells will become faulty in their turn.

Using stem cells to rebuild the immune system is currently a last option when other treatments for severe arthritis have not been

effective. Rebuilding the immune system is very different from using stem cells to regenerate cartilage, which is relatively safe though technically extremely complex.

The genetic approach

The study of genes and the practice of gene therapy is often heralded as the future direction of research into rheumatic diseases and the opening of a door to a new age of treatment.

The theory is that the analysis of an individual's genes will reveal the biological factors that drive his or her arthritis. At the same time, it will allow an evaluation of the person's potential responses to specific drugs, whether they are disease-modifiers or biological agents. Equipped with this unique, individualized information, medical scientists and healthcare professionals would be able to devise a tailor-made treatment.

However, this approach has so far borne little fruit. The expense of analysing a person's genes and developing a drug regime that will probably benefit only one person is not an attractive proposition for a pharmaceutical company used to making sizeable profits. Yet this individualized treatment is almost certain to happen one day, but no-one knows when it will become routine. It is most likely to benefit us in the distant future.

GENOME RESEARCH
A fully automated gene production line uses a robot and a computer vision system to select and deliver particular sequences of DNA that enable scientists to investigate an individual's genes.

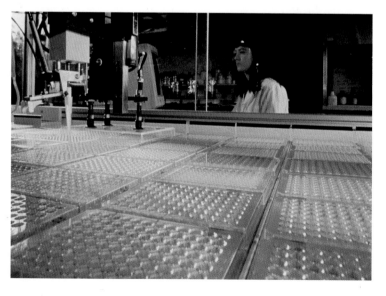

Improvements in surgery

Techniques and materials for joint replacement surgery continue to improve and the effectiveness of treatment is constantly being evaluated. In one line of research, medical scientists are investigating the reasons why artificial joints fail in certain people after a relatively short time. They are endeavouring to identify biological markers that could predict which individuals are more likely to be susceptible to infection or to the premature loosening of an implant.

Researchers are also examining ways of developing better types of cement for joint replacements in the knee and hip. In addition, advances in imaging techniques to study joints may result in better designs for implants as well as more efficient surgery.

Q&A

If I take part in trials of a new drug, does this mean I can get the latest treatment and what are the risks?

Taking part in a clinical trial does not guarantee access to new drugs because some participants have to receive the standard treatment. Drug trials are never entirely free of risk as the new medications, although they have been subjected to rigorous tests, may have unexpected side-effects. However, we all want treatments to be tried and tested and so we all need to support trials.

How you can help with research

If you have arthritis there are ways you can contribute to research. Doctors and scientists need your personal experience to help them build up databanks of information.

Thousands of people volunteer to participate in clinical trials, in which new or revised treatments are clinically tested on people, then monitored for effectiveness and long-term safety.

These carefully controlled trials require a degree of commitment as they can extend for two or three years, or even longer. Remember, too, that for the duration of the trial, you may have to discontinue taking any drugs that you are currently prescribed, which could mean your arthritis is less well controlled. If you feel you may be a suitable candidate for a drug trial, ask your doctor or specialist for information and advice.

Participating in surveys

You can help medical researchers by taking part in surveys to collect data from people with arthritis on such issues as pain, disability, side-effects of medication, and lifestyle. Your information will be treated as strictly confidential and will be of great value to health professionals; there is a good chance that it may eventually benefit yourself and others with arthritis by leading to improved care and treatment.

Researchers are also experimenting with the possibility of using stem cell transplants to repair cartilage damaged by osteoarthritis.

Glossary

Acute Term to describe a symptom or condition that comes on suddenly.

Analgesic A drug that relieves pain.

Antibody A protein in the blood that destroys substances or organisms that may be harmful to the body.

Anti-inflammatories Drugs, such as corticosteroids and NSAIDs, that reduce inflammation.

Antioxidants Chemicals that can neutralize free radicals.

Autoimmune Term to describe a condition in which the body attacks its own tissues.

Chronic Term to describe a symptom (e.g. pain) or condition (e.g. arthritis) that lasts for a long time and is slow to change.

Collagen Strong protein that forms part of cartilage and bone.

Corticosteroids Drugs that reduce inflammation by suppressing allergic responses and the immune system.

Cytokine Chemical that stimulates the immune system to combat infection.

Endorphins (encephalins) Chemicals produced by the brain and central nervous system to relieve the pain.

Enthesitis Inflammation at the point where a tendon is attached to bone.

Enzymes Proteins that increase the rate of chemical reactions in the cells of the body.

Erythrocyte Red blood cell.

Essential fatty acid Polyunsaturated fatty acids, such as omega-3, that the body needs but cannot make.

Free radicals Naturally occurring molecules that can harm the body's tissues and damage DNA, causing various health problems.

Holistic Term that describes treatment of the whole person rather than just the symptoms.

Hormone Chemical with a specific function that is released directly into the bloodstream by a gland (e.g. adrenal gland) or a tissue (e.g. kidney, brain, or intestine).

Leukocyte White blood cell.

Magnetic resonance imaging A diagnostic technique that uses high-frequency radio waves to scan the internal structures of the body, especially the nervous system.

Marker Chemical or gene that indicates, but does not necessarily confirm, the presence of a condition or disorder.

Metabolism Term that describes all the chemical reactions in the body, especially those that form new substances, release energy, or detoxify foreign chemicals.

Mind–body therapies Techniques and approaches that harness thoughts, feelings, imagination, and actions in order to influence a person's biochemical and structural processes.

NSAIDs Non-steroidal anti-inflammatory drugs that relieve painful inflammation and stiffness in muscles, joints, and bones.

Prostaglandins Synthetic or naturally occurring chemicals that can contract muscles, inflame damaged tissue, lower blood pressure, or produce mucus in the lining of the stomach.

Range of motion The normal amount that a joint can be moved in certain directions.

Supplements Nutrients, such as vitamins, minerals, and trace elements, which can be taken to supplement the diet.

Synovium The cartilage lining of a joint which produces synovial fluid.

Tendinitis Inflammation of a tendon.

Tenosynovitis Swelling of a tendon and the synovial membrane of a joint.

Topical Applied to the skin.

Trace element A mineral (e.g. zinc, copper, and selenium) which the body needs in tiny amounts and can only get from digesting food.

Ultrasound A diagnostic technique that uses high-frequency sound waves to scan internal structures of the body and to treat injuries of the soft tissues.

Unsaturated fat (including polyunsaturated fat) Fat that contains fatty acids but no cholesterol.

Useful addressses

Arthritis Care
18 Stephenson Way,
London NW1 2HD
Tel: 020 7380 6500
Helpline: 0808 800 4050 (Mon–Fri
10am–4pm)
Fax: 020 7380 6505
Email: helplines@arthritiscare.org.uk
Website: www.arthritiscare.org.uk

Arthritis Ireland
1 Clanwilliam Square,
Grand Canal Quay, Dublin 2
Tel: (01) 661 8188
Fax: (01) 661 8261
Website: www.arthritis-foundation.com
Email: info@arthritisireland.ie

Arthritis Research Campaign
Copeman House, St Mary's Court,
St Mary's Gate, Chesterfield,
Derbyshire S41 7TD
Tel: 0870 850 5000 or 01246 558033
Fax: 01246 558007
Website: www.arc.org.uk

Arthritis Australia
1st Floor, 52 Parramatta Road,
Forest Lodge, NSW 2037
GPO Box 121 Sydney NSW 2001
Freecall in Australia: 1800 111 101
Tel: (02) 9552 6085
Fax: (02) 9552 6078
Email: info@arthritisaustralia.com.au
Website: www.arthritisaustralia.com.au

Australian Rheumatology Association
145 Macquarie Street,
Sydney NSW 2000
Tel: (02) 92565458
Email: robynm@racp.edu.au
Website: www.rheumatology.org.au

British Association for Counselling and Psychotherapy
BACP House, 35–37 Albert Street,
Rugby, Warks CV21 2SG
Tel: 0870 443 5252
Fax: 0870 443 5161
Email: bacp@bacp.co.uk
Website: www.bacp.co.uk

British Society for Rheumatology
Bride House, 18–20 Bride Lane,
London EC4Y 8EE
Tel: 020 7842 0900
Fax: 020 7842 0901
Email: bsr@rheumatology.org.uk
Website: www.rheumatology.org.uk

The Chartered Society of Physiotherapy
14 Bedford Row, London WC1R 4ED
Tel: 020 7306 6666
Website: www.csp.org.uk

College of Occupational Therapists
106–114 Borough High Street,
Southwark, London SE1 1LB
Tel: 020 7357 6480
Website: www.cot.org.uk

Disabled Living Foundation
380–384 Harrow Road,
London W9 2HU
Tel: 020 7289 6111
Helpline: 0845 130 9177
Email: info@dlf.org.uk
Website: www.dlf.org.uk

Help the Aged
207–221 Pentonville Road,
London N1 9UZ
Tel: 020 7278 1114
Fax: 020 7278 1116
Email: info@helptheaged
Website: www.helptheaged.org.uk

Specific conditions
BackCare
16 Elmtree Road,
Teddington, Middlesex TW11 8ST
Tel: 020 8977 5474
Fax: 020 8943 5318
Email: info@backcare.org.uk
Website: www.backcare.org.uk

British Sjögren's Syndrome Association
PO Box 10867, Birmingham B16 0ZW
Tel: 0121 455 6532
Fax : 0121 455 6532
Email: kate@bssa.uk.net
Website: www.bssa.uk.net

Fibromyalgia Association
PO Box 206, Stourbridge,
West Midlands DY9 8YL
Helpline: 0870 220 1232
Fax: 0870 752 5118
Email: fmauk@hotmail.com
Website: www.fibromyalgia-associationuk.org

Lupus UK
St James House, Eastern Road,
Romford, Essex RM1 3NH
Tel: 01708 731251
Fax: 01708 731252
Email: headoffice@lupusuk.org.uk
Website: www.lupusuk.com

National Ankylosing Spondylitis Society
PO Box 179, Mayfield,
East Sussex TN20 6ZL
Tel: 01435 873527
Fax: 01435 873027
Email: nass@nass.co.uk
Website: www.nass.co.uk

National Osteoporosis Society
Camerton, Bath BA2 0PJ
Tel: 01761 471771
Fax: 01761 471104
Email: info@nos.org.uk
Website: www.nos.org.uk

National Rheumatoid Arthritis Society
Unit B4 Westacott Business Centre
Westacott Way, Littlewick Green
Maidenhead, Berkshire SL6 3RT
Tel: 01628 823524
Helpline: 0845 458 3969
Fax: 0845 458 3971
Email: enquiries@rheumatoid.org.uk
Website: www.rheumatoid.org.uk

Psoriatic Arthropathy Alliance
PO Box 111,
St Albans, Herts AL2 3JQ
Tel: 0870 770 3212
Fax: 0870 770 3213
Website: www.thepaa.org

The RSI Association
PO Box 700,
Southampton SO17 1LQ
Tel: 023 8058 4314
Fax: 023 8055 6902
Email: rsia@keytools.com
Website: www.rsi.org.uk

The Scleroderma Society
3 Caple Road, London NW10 8AB
Tel: 020 8961 4912
Email: info@sclerodermasociety.co.uk
www.sclerodermasociety.co.uk

Complementary therapies

Association of Physical & Natural Therapists
27 Old Gloucester Street,
London WC1N 3XX
Tel: 0845 345 2345
Email: info@apnt.org
Website: www.apnt.org

British Acupuncture Council
63 Jeddo Road, London W12 9HQ
Tel: 020 8735 0400
Fax: 020 8735 0404
Email: info@acupuncture.org.uk
Website: www.acupuncture.org.uk

The British Chiropractic Association
Blagrave House, 17 Blagrave Street,
Reading, Berkshire RG1 1QB
Tel: 0118 950 5950
Email: enquiries@chiropractic-uk.co.uk
Website: www.chiropractic-uk.co.uk

British Complementary Medicine Association
PO Box 5122,
Bournemouth BH8 0WG
Tel: 0845 3455977
Email: info@bcma.co.uk
Website: www.bcma.co.uk

British Medical Acupuncture Society
BMAS House,
3 Winnington Court,
Northwich, Cheshire CW8 1AQ
Tel: 01606 786782
Fax: 01606 786783
Email: admin@medical-acupuncture.org.uk
Website: www.medical-acupuncture.co.uk

British Osteopathy Association
Langham House West, Mill Street,
Luton, Bedfordshire LU1 2NA
Tel: 01582 488455
Fax: 01582 481533
Email: enquiries@osteopathy.org
Website: www.osteopathy.org

The British School of Osteopathy
275 Borough High Street,
London SE1 1JE
Tel: 020 7407 0222
Fax: 020 7089 5300
Website: www.bso.ac.uk

The Feldenkrais Guild UK
Tel: 07000 785506
Email: enq@feldenkrais.co.uk
Website: www.feldenkrais.co.uk

International Federation of Professional Aromatherapists
82 Ashby Road, Hinckley,
Leicestershire LE10 1SN
Tel: 01455 637987
Email: admin@IFPAroma.org
Website: www.ifparoma.org

International Institute of Reflexology (UK)
146 Upperthorpe, Walkley,
Sheffield S6 3NF
Tel/Fax: 01142 812100
E-mail: info@reflexology-uk.net
Website: www.reflexology-uk.co.uk

National Institute of Medical Herbalists
Elm House, 54 Mary Arches Street,
Exeter EX4 3BA
Tel: 01392 426022
Fax: 01392 498963
Email: nimh@ukexeter.freeserve.co.uk
Website: www.nimh.org.uk

The PILATESfoundation® UK Ltd
PO Box 36052, London SW16 1XQ
Tel: 07071 781 859
Fax: 020 7489 0403
Website: www.pilatesfoundation.com

Society of Homeopaths
11 Brookfield, Duncan Close,
Moulton Park, Northants NN3 6WL
Tel: 0845 450 6611
Fax: 0845 450 6622
Web: www.homeopathy-soh.org

**The Society of Teachers of the
Alexander Technique**
1st Floor, Linton House,
39–51 Highgate Road,
London NW5 1RS
Tel: 0845 230 7828
Fax: 020 7482 5435
Email: office@stat.org.uk
Website: www.stat.org.uk

Tai Chi Finder Ltd
21 The Avenue, London E11 2EE
Tel: 0845 8900744
Website: www.taichifinder.co.uk

Trager UK
Tel: 01903 717987
Email: Richard.tilbrook@tiscali.co.uk
Website: www.trager.co.uk

Yoga Village UK
Website: www.yogauk.com

Pain
Action on Pain
20 Necton Road, Little Dunham,
Norfolk PE32 2DN
Tel/Fax: 01760 725993
Painline: 0845 6031593
Email: info@action-on-pain.co.uk
Website: www.action-on-pain.co.uk

British Pain Society
21 Portland Place, London W1B 1PY
Tel: 020 7631 8870
Fax: 020 7323 2015
Email: info@britishpainsociety.org
Website: www.britishpainsociety.org

Pain Association Scotland
Cramond House,
Cramond Glebe Road,
Edinburgh EH4 6NS
Tel: 0131 3127955
Fax: 0131 3126007
Freephone: 0800 7836059
Email: info@painassociation.com
Website: www.painassociation.com

Pain Concern
PO Box 13256, Haddington,
Edinburgh EH41 4YD
Tel: 01620 822572
Fax: 01620 829138
E-mail: info@painconcern.org.uk
Website: www.painconcern.org.uk

The Pain Relief Foundation
Clinical Sciences Centre,
University Hospital Aintree,
Lower Lane, Liverpool L9 7AL
Tel: 0151 529 5820
Fax: 0151 529 5821
Email: secretary@painrelieffoundation.org.uk
Website: www.painrelieffoundation.org.uk

**Tame the Pain (for specialized pain
clinics in the UK)**
Website: www.tamethepain.co.uk

Children
**Children's Chronic Arthritis
Association**
47 Battenhall Avenue,
Worcester WR5 2HN
Tel: 01905 763556
Website: www.ccaa.org.uk

The Children's Hospital School,
GOS Hospital for Children
Great Ormond Street,
London WC1N 3JH
Tel 020 7813 8269
Email: mjlgos@aol.com
Website: www.schoolsite.edex.net.uk/262

**Choices for Families of Children
with Arthritis**
PO Box 58, Hove, BN3 5WN
Website: www.kidswitharthritis.org

Contact a Family
209–211 City Road,
London EC1V 1JN
Helpline: 0808 808 3555 (Mon–Fri
10am–4pm)
Tel: 0207 608 8700
Email: info@cafamily.org
Website: www.cafamily.org.uk

**Give Rheumatoid Arthritis Children
Encouragement (GRACE)**
50 Wood Street, St Annes FY8 1QG
Tel: 01253 720303
Fax: 01253 728070
Website: www.fyldecoast.co.uk/grace

**National Association of Special
Educational Needs**
4–5 Amber Business Village,
Amber Close, Amington,
Tamworth B77 4RP
Tel: 01827 311500
Email: welcome@nasen.org.uk
Website: www.nasen.org.uk

**Present (formerly the National
Association for the Education of
Sick Children)**
18 Victoria Park Square,
London E2 9PF
Tel: 020 8980 8523
Email: naesc@ednsick.demon.co.uk
Website: www.sickchildren.org.uk

Index

About the authors

Arthritis Care is the largest UK-wide voluntary organisation working for people with arthritis and has around 70,000 supporters. Arthritis Care runs a confidential helpline service and publishes a range of information publications on all aspects of living with arthritis, including a bi-monthly magazine. It campaigns for greater understanding of the needs of people with arthritis and runs Arthritis Care Awareness Week every year. It also runs a range of self-management courses and helps put people in touch with others who are affected by the condition.

David L Scott is Professor of Clinical Rheumatology at King's College Hospital, London. **Howard Bird** is Professor of Pharmacological Rheumatology at the University of Leeds. **Andrew Hamer** is Consultant Orthopaedic Surgeon at the Northern General Hospital, Sheffield. **Alison Hammond** is Senior Lecturer in Rheumatology at the University of Brighton and Rheumatology Research Therapist in Derby. **Mike Hurley** is Reader in Physiotherapy at King's College London. **Dorothy Pattison** is Lecturer in Dietetics at the University of Plymouth. **Janet Harkess** is Clinical Specialist Occupational Therapist based in Fife. **Paula Jeffreson** is a Specialist Occupational Therapist in Rheumatology based in Shropshire. **Caroline Green** is a freelance health writer with a special interest in arthritis and complementary therapies.

Acknowledgments

Dorling Kindersley would like to thank the following: Christine Edwards, Kate Llewelyn, Jo Cumming and the Helpline team at Arthritis Care for their expert review and advice on content and usability. Ann Baggaley for her invaluable contribution to the sections: Looking After Your Arthritis, Eating to Ease Arthritis, The Outlook for Arthritis, and Arthritis in the Future, and for proofreading. The Food Standards Agency for help with the information on salt and fat labelling, and on the alcoholic content of some drinks. Ruth Jenkinson for new photography. Pat Perse-White and Ann Greenhouse for modelling. Roisin Donaghy for hair and make-up. Hilary Bird for the index.

Picture credits